Beginner's Guide to

Crystals

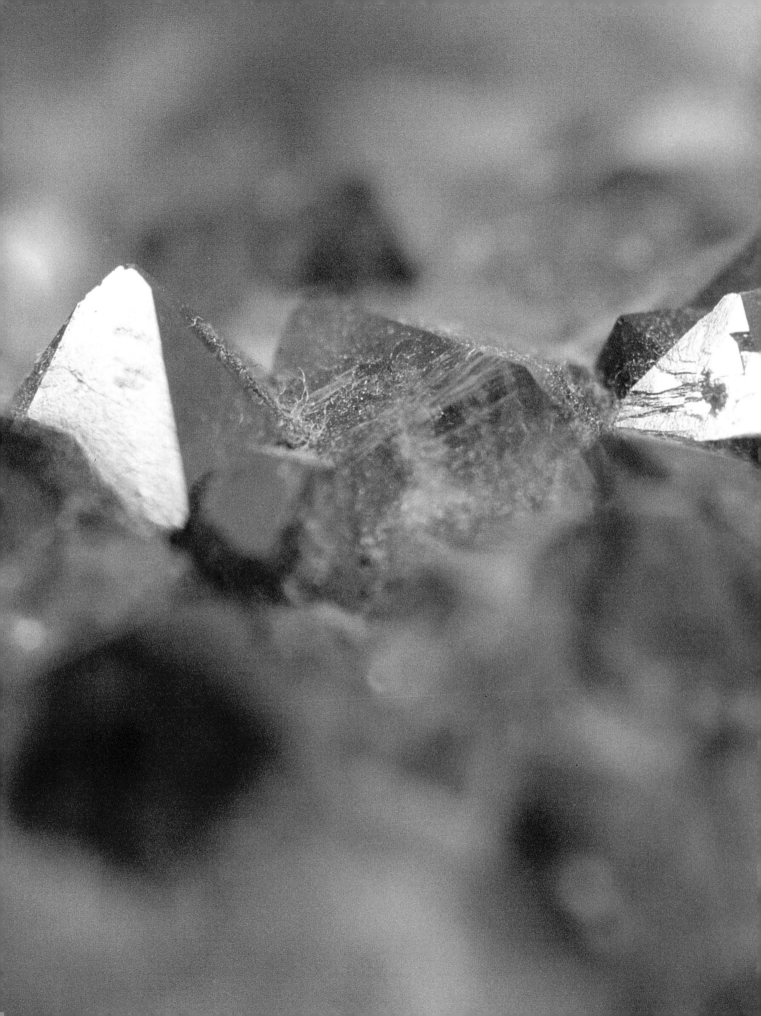

BEGINNER'S GUIDE TO
CRYSTALS

Denise Whichello Brown

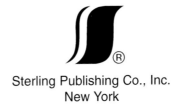

Sterling Publishing Co., Inc.
New York

Creative director: Sarah King
Editor: Clare Haworth-Maden
Project editor: Sally MacEachern
Designer: 2H Design

Library of Congress Cataloging-in-Publication Data Available

10   9   8   7   6   5   4   3   2   1

Published in 2003 by Sterling Publishing Co., Inc.
387 Park Avenue South, New York, N.Y. 10016

This book was designed and produced by
D&S Books Ltd
Kerswell, Parkham Ash
Bideford, Devon, EX39 5PR

Distributed in Canada by Sterling Publishing
c/o Canadian Manda Group,
One Atlantic Avenue, Suite 105
Toronto, Ontario, Canada M6K 3E7

Printed in China

ISBN 1-4027-1010-0

CONTENTS

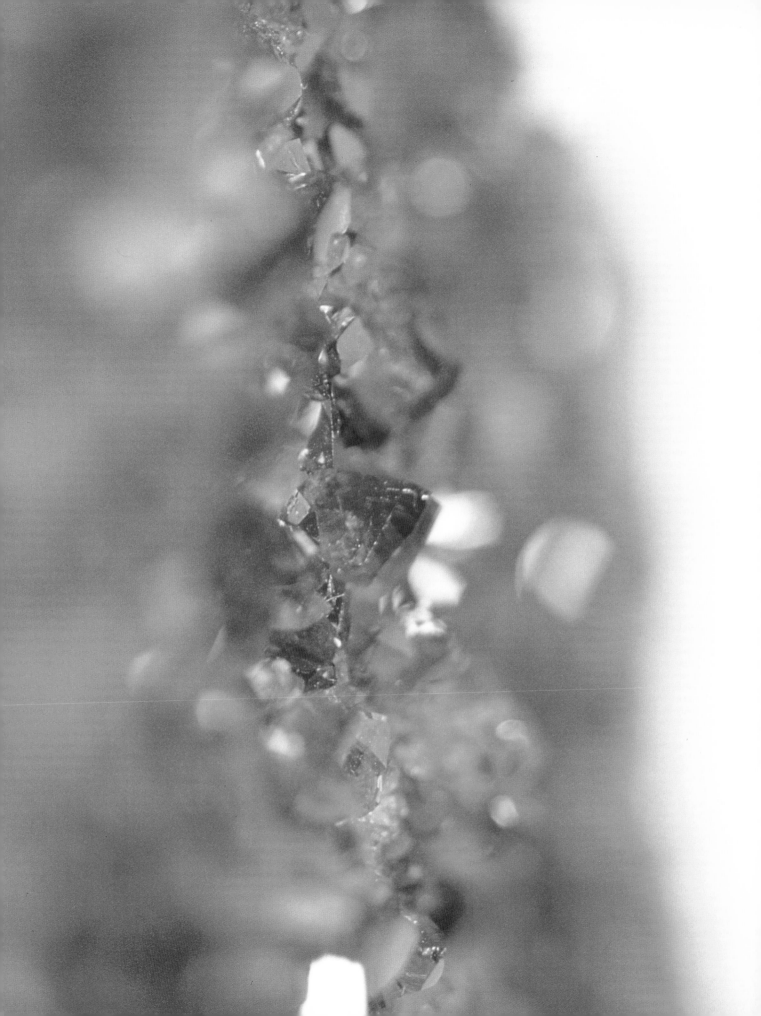

Crystal healing (which is sometimes referred to as crystal, or gem, therapy) is the use of crystals and stones for therapeutic and healing purposes.

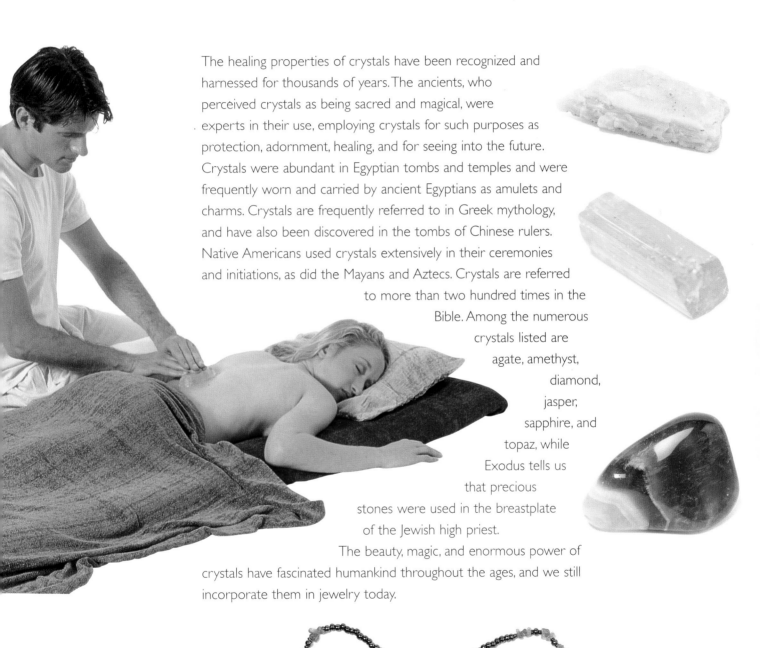

The healing properties of crystals have been recognized and harnessed for thousands of years. The ancients, who perceived crystals as being sacred and magical, were experts in their use, employing crystals for such purposes as protection, adornment, healing, and for seeing into the future. Crystals were abundant in Egyptian tombs and temples and were frequently worn and carried by ancient Egyptians as amulets and charms. Crystals are frequently referred to in Greek mythology, and have also been discovered in the tombs of Chinese rulers. Native Americans used crystals extensively in their ceremonies and initiations, as did the Mayans and Aztecs. Crystals are referred to more than two hundred times in the Bible. Among the numerous crystals listed are agate, amethyst, diamond, jasper, sapphire, and topaz, while Exodus tells us that precious stones were used in the breastplate of the Jewish high priest. The beauty, magic, and enormous power of crystals have fascinated humankind throughout the ages, and we still incorporate them in jewelry today.

Wearing stones is a highly effective way to promote health and healing.

In this book you will discover how to select and use crystals for a multitude of purposes in your everyday life. The healing properties of specific stones are detailed fully to enable you to help yourself attain physical, mental, emotional, and spiritual healing. Offering the ability to enhance and perhaps change your life, the many benefits of crystal healing include:

✳ relief from stress and tension

✳ endowing the work or home environment with peace and tranquillity

✳ protection against unwanted energies

✳ the transformation of negative into positive energies

✳ enhanced meditative powers and a reconnection with the spiritual realms

✳ the attraction of abundance and an aiding of manifestation

✳ the attraction of love

✳ a healing ability on every level, rejuvenating the whole being—body, mind, and spirit

✳ the amplification of healing abilities

✳ stimulation of the mind, enhancing creativity and the development of new ideas

✳ the gift of energy and vitality

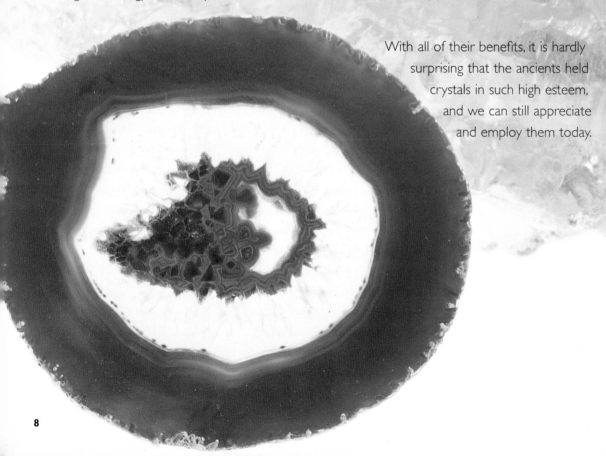

With all of their benefits, it is hardly surprising that the ancients held crystals in such high esteem, and we can still appreciate and employ them today.

The
Configuration
of
Crystals

The Configuration of Crystals

The generally accepted definition of a crystal is a solid substance with a geometrically regular shape. The name "crystal" comes from the Greek *Krystallos*, meaning "ice," because the Greeks believed that rock crystal was water that had been frozen forever by the gods. It was not until 1784 that a French mineralogist, René-Just Haüy (who accidentally dropped one and discovered that the fragments all displayed a similar appearance), published his theory on the structure of crystals.

Crystals are available in many shapes and forms. You can purchase rough stones in their natural state or polished stones that have been tumbled in large, rotating drums filled with water, fine sand then being added to polish them further, a process that takes a few weeks. Both unpolished, natural stones and polished ones provide the same beneficial healing energies.

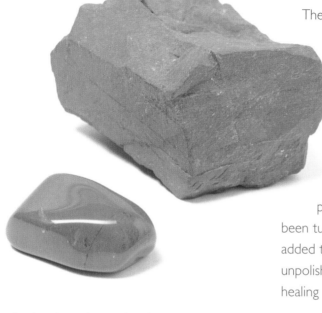

Rough and smooth examples of red jasper.

Clusters

When several crystals have grown together in a cluster, they are referred to as "groups." Clusters are often placed in rooms to change the energy of the environment and to cleanse and transform negativity into positive energy. The amethyst cluster illustrated is a wonderful transformer of negative energies that can be used to cleanse and activate other crystals, as well as rooms. A cluster is recommended in the work environment to deflect other people's stress, tension, and frustration from you and to draw harmony toward you.

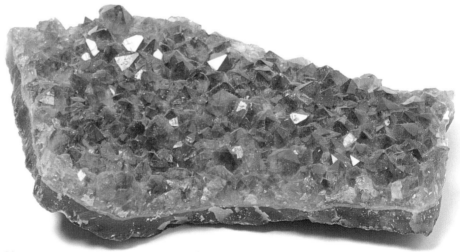

Amethyst cluster.

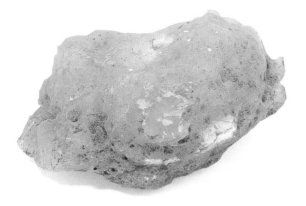

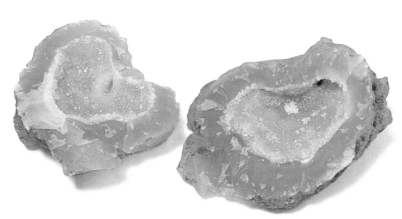

Chalcedony geode.

Geodes

A geode is produced when a group of crystals grows together to fill a small hollow or cyst. Geodes vary enormously in size and shape. They have a womblike appearance and bring protection, healing, and spiritual growth. The one illustrated here is of blue chalcedony, which is particularly effective for enhancing communication and inspiration, as well as providing protection for the very sensitive.

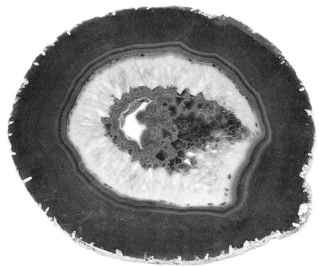

Slices

Sometimes a stone may be cut into slices so that its beauty is revealed. Crystal slices are an ideal aid to meditation and may also be placed in a room or on the body for healing purposes. This slice of blue agate encourages calmness and contemplation, gently dissolving tension and anxiety.

Doughnuts

Slice of blue agate.

A doughnut is a round stone with a hole in it. Turquoise doughnuts are commonly carved in Nepal and India, but natural doughnuts are found occasionally. They are ideal for meditation, for gazing into other dimensions. They may also be used to draw energy toward you and to clear a blocked chakra. Natural stones with holes in them have always been thought to bring luck.

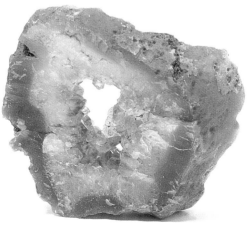

Amethyst doughnut.

Eggs

Crystals may be fashioned into egg shapes. Such stones fit perfectly into the hand and are ideal for meditation. Their smooth shape and texture makes them perfect for massage to relieve blockages, while the pointed end can be used for such therapies as reflexology and acupressure.

The three eggs illustrated are brecciated jasper, grossularite (a type of garnet), and rhodonite. Brecciated jasper—a wonderful conglomerate of rust red, brown, pink, gray, and cream—is excellent for grounding, both physically and emotionally. A powerful healer of the liver and gallbladder, it may also be placed under the pillow to assist dream recall. The green grossularite egg promotes healing, particularly of the heart. The beautiful rose-pink, rhodonite egg is a stone of love that activates the heart chakra, filling it with the purity of unconditional love.

Crystal Balls

Crystal balls or spheres may either be natural or fabricated. They are used to gaze into the past or future or to evaluate a current situation (see the section on scrying, page 47).

Pyramids

Pyramid-shaped crystals focus and amplify energy through their apex. They are often used to charge and preserve objects.

Single-terminated Crystal

A single-terminated crystal has one flat end and one pointed, or terminated, end, with energy being focused within the terminated end. Such crystals are mainly used for healing and meditation. The healing energies are concentrated through the point of the crystal.

Single-terminated crystal.

Double-terminated Crystal

A double-terminated crystal has a point at both ends, enabling energy to move in one or both directions and to be transmitted, or drawn in, through both ends. Such crystals may be used for healing, placed under the pillow to encourage dreams, or carried to provide protection.

Less Common Crystals

Barnacle Crystal

A barnacle crystal is a crystal that is covered, or partly covered, with smaller crystals. Such crystals are said to be teaching crystals, the large crystal being said to be the teacher, or "old soul," to whose knowledge the smaller crystals have been attracted.

Bridge Crystal

A bridge crystal is a small crystal that penetrates a larger crystal. Such a crystal may be useful in times of change or in meditation, when trying to make a link with other dimensions and universes. It acts not only as a bridge between the self and other worlds, but as a bridge between the self and others, making it useful for teaching purposes.

Channeling Crystal

A channeling crystal has a seven-sided face on the front of the crystal's terminated end and a triangular face on the opposite side (back) of the terminated end. Such a crystal may be employed for channeling information, truth, and wisdom from the spiritual realms.

Elestial or El Crystal

The elestial or el crystal can be recognized by its natural terminations and the growth of smaller crystals over the body and face of an etched, or multilayered, crystal. It can sometimes look as though one crystal has grown over another or candle wax has dripped onto the crystal.

Elestials activate the third eye, remove negative energy blocks, balance the male and female energies, and assist with meditation. It is said that they carry the memory of all that existed prior to humanity. While meditating, hold the elestial in one hand and use the index finger of your other hand to bring forth the wisdom of the knowledge of the universe. You may also be able to access past lives and gain an understanding of the lessons that have to be learned in this life, as well as in future lives.

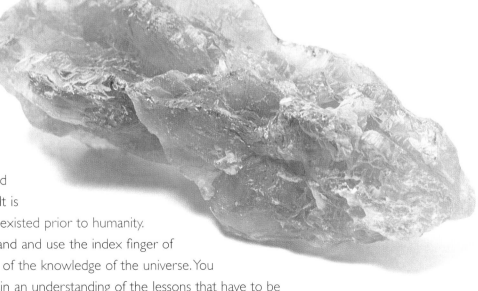

Elestial crystal.

Manifestation Crystal

The rather rare manifestation crystal is a small crystal that is totally enclosed by a larger crystal. Such a crystal may be used for manifesting the highest good.

Phantom Crystal

A phantom crystal can be recognized by its namesake "phantom," an image of the structure of another crystal (whose outline may either be partial or complete) within the crystal. Phantom crystals are useful for spiritual development.

Record-keeper Crystal

A record-keeper crystal may be recognized by one or more raised triangles on one or two faces. Ancient wisdom and secrets are said to be stored within these crystals, and some believe that the Atlanteans and Lemurians purposely programed them. The record-keeper crystal may be used in meditation to gain access to ancient knowledge.

Twin Crystal

The twin crystal can be recognized when two crystals have grown together. This crystal can be useful when two people are either working together or in a relationship.

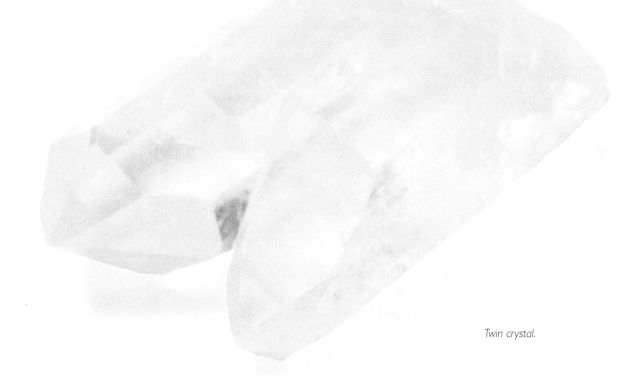

Twin crystal.

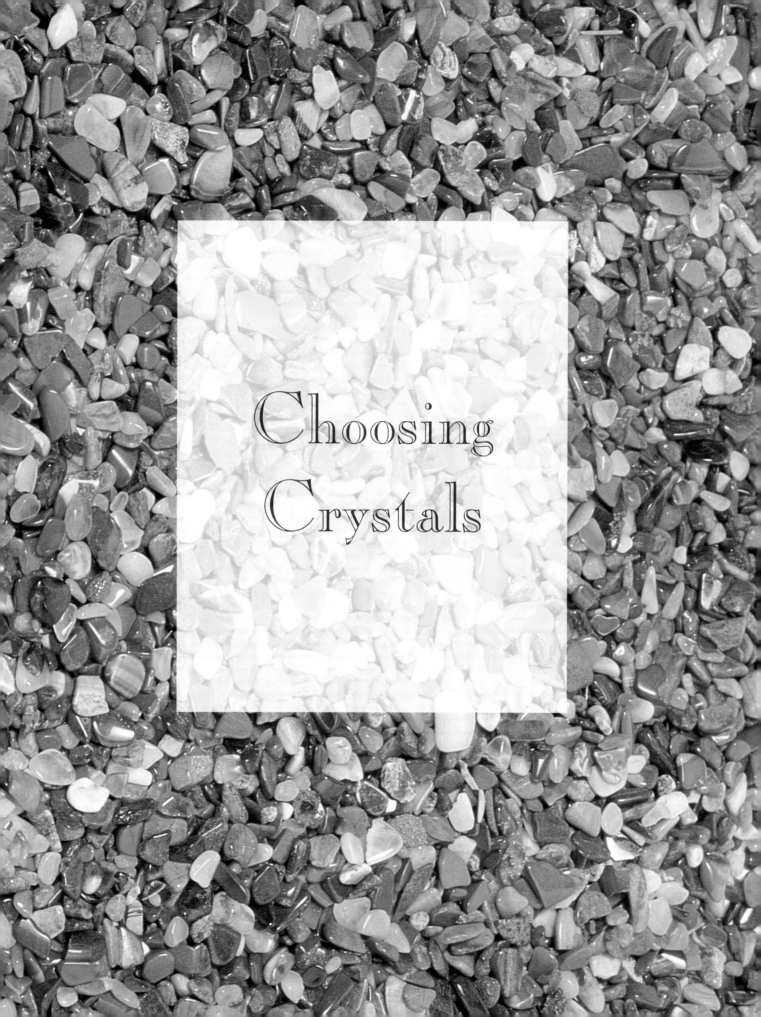

Choosing
Crystals

Choosing Crystals

There are no rules or regulations to abide by when selecting crystals: the stones that you choose may be large, small, uncut, polished, clear, or colored. Your instinct will guide you to the stone that will help you the most. Always follow your intuition: if you trust in your feelings, you can be sure that the crystal that you are drawn to is the right one for you at this time in your life. Do not listen to other people's advice—a particular stone may look or feel good to them, but that doesn't mean that it is the right one for you. Follow your instinct!

If a crystal is meant for you, you will feel an immediate attraction to it. It's rather like meeting a stranger for the first time and having an immediate response to them, be it a feeling of strong antipathy or a more neutral or disinterested feeling. You may not be able to explain why in rational or logical terms, but simply sense inside whether or not you are on the same wavelength. It's exactly the same with stones. All crystals vibrate on a particular frequency, just as human beings do, and the crystals that will appeal to you the most will be those that vibrate on a similar frequency to your own and that are the most beneficial to you at this particular stage in your progression.

"Finding" your crystals should be a magical and joyous experience, whether you acquire them from New Age stores, forests, mountains, or ancient sites or receive one as a gift. My most treasured stones are those that I either unearthed myself, for instance, at Mount Sinai in Egypt, or those that friends unearthed and then gave to me.

Do not assume that the crystals that "find" you and that are right for you today will always be the most effective ones for you. Crystals sometimes need to move on. If you feel an overpowering urge to pass a crystal on to a friend, follow your instinct in the knowledge that the crystal has completed its work with you, and let it go willingly and with love. A new crystal will very quickly "find" you! Do not become too attached to a particular stone because suddenly losing a crystal is a very common experience. If this happens to you, do not become too distressed: it is an indication that the crystal has served its purpose and that it is time for you both to move on.

If a crystal is attuned to your vibration, it will communicate with you. You may experience all sorts of inexplicable sensations while choosing a crystal, including the following:

* heat emanating from the crystal

* cold energy

* a sudden burst of energy that may feel like an electric charge

* tingling in your fingers

* a pulsing or vibration

* an inner knowledge

* a feeling of balance and wholeness

* a wave of heat permeating your body

* warmth in your heart

* an overwhelming sensation of love

* perfume emanating from the crystal

* colors surrounding the crystal

* a flash of light from the crystal

* a moistness in your hands

* the crystal apparently "jumping" out at you or falling at your feet

* a sudden rush of excitement

* a protective feeling

* an urge to laugh

* shivers down your spine

* a light-headed sensation

* a sound in your ears

* changes in your breathing

* the knowledge that you have just *got* to have it!

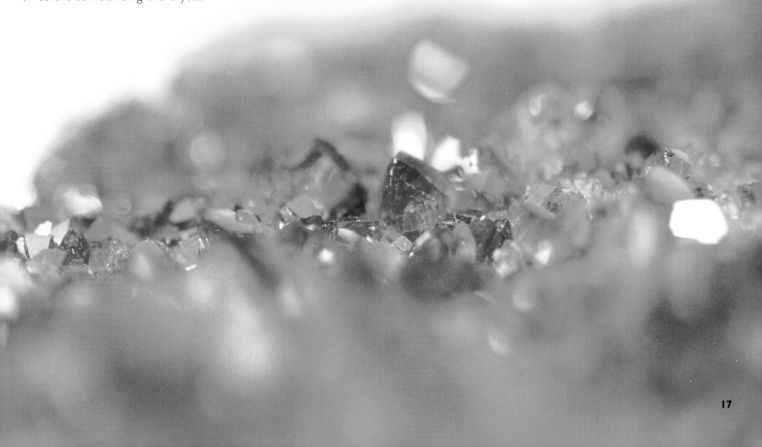

Methods of Choosing Crystals

Although individual methods of choosing crystals vary from person to person, you may find the following useful.

1. Choosing With Your Eyes

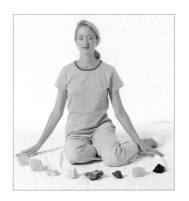

a) Spread out the crystals in front of you. Close your eyes and take a few deep breaths to clear your mind.

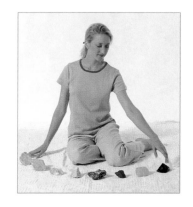

b) Now open your eyes very quickly and pick up the first crystal that catches your eye.

c) Your choice of crystal will not necessarily be the most beautiful, the biggest, or the most expensive stone. The one that attracts your attention will be in attunement with you.

2. Scanning

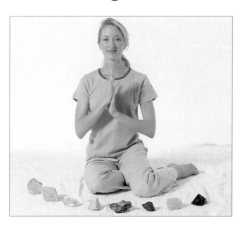

a) Begin by shaking out your hands to release any blocked energy. Briskly rub the palms of your hands together to concentrate energy into them and increase your sensitivity.

b) Close your eyes and take a few deep breaths to clear any negativity from your body and mind.

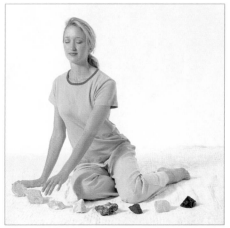

c) Very slowly run your hand over all of the stones without opening your eyes. If you are right-handed, use your left hand, and if you are left-handed, use your right hand. Do you feel any of the sensations described on page 17, such as heat, cold energy, or tingling? At least one crystal should draw you to it like a magnet. Another common perception is that one particular stone feels "sticky"—if so, this is the stone that you should select.

3. Vibration

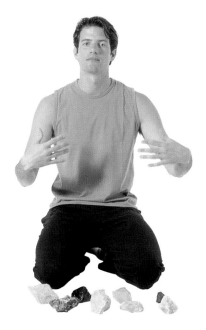

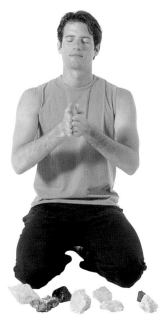

a) Shake out your hands to release any blocked energy.

b) Vigorously rub the palms of your hands together to sensitize them. Take a few deep breaths to calm your mind and increase your focus.

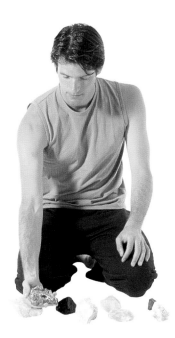

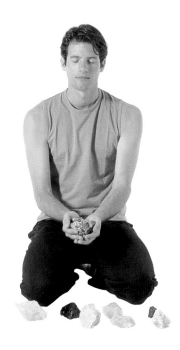

c) Pick up each crystal one by one, sensing any vibrations. Use your left hand if you are right-handed, and your right hand if you are left-handed, to receive any information.

d) If the vibration of any particular crystal resonates with you, that is the stone that is right for you.

4. Using a Pendulum

Using a pendulum is both very easy and an excellent way of enhancing your intuition. A pendulum is usually a crystal suspended on a chain, although some may be made of wood or metal. They are readily available in New Age stores, but you could also suspend an everyday object, such as a key or a ring, from a piece of string or a leather thong.

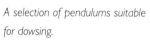

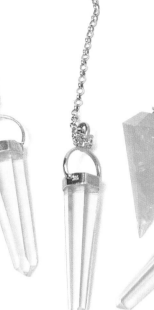

A handmade pendulum will enable you to choose the crystal that is meant for you.

A selection of pendulums suitable for dowsing.

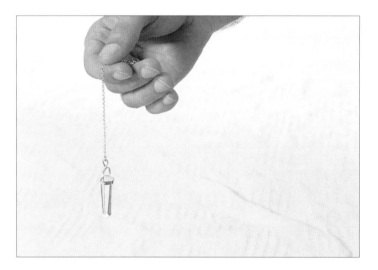

a) Gently hold your pendulum between your thumb and index finger as illustrated. Do not grasp the chain too tightly and make sure that your neck and shoulders are free from tension.

b) Either mentally or aloud, ask your pendulum which movement indicates a "yes" answer. (The pendulum will usually swing either clockwise or counterclockwise to indicate "yes.") To check your pendulum's accuracy, ask it one or more questions to which the answer is definitely "yes," such as, "My name is . . . is that correct?"

c) Wait until the pendulum has stopped moving and then, either mentally or aloud, ask it which movement indicates "no." Note which way the pendulum swings.

d) In the same way, establish which movement indicates "don't know." (This will often be from side to side or up and down.) Make a note of your pendulum's responses for future reference.

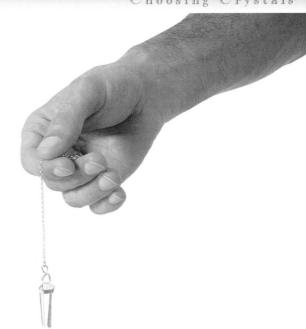

Holding a pendulum correctly.

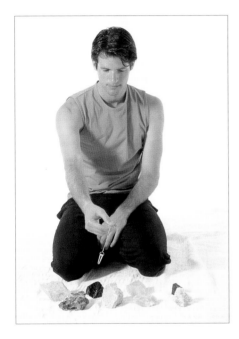

e) Now hold your pendulum over each crystal in turn and ask a question like "Is this crystal right for me?" or "Is this crystal suitable for healing/meditation?"

f) If you are dowsing over a large number of crystals, pass the pendulum very slowly over the top of all of the crystals to see if the pendulum starts to react above any particular stone. Return to any "reactive" stones and ask a question while suspending the pendulum directly above them.

g) You may also choose a crystal for a friend using a pendulum. To do this, follow the same procedure but, as you hold the pendulum over each crystal, ask "Is this crystal suitable for . . .?"

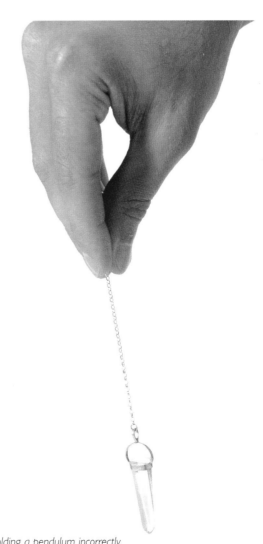

Holding a pendulum incorrectly.

5. Kinesiology

Kinesiology, or muscle-testing, which involves working with a partner, is another method of choosing crystals. Kinesiology's amazing accuracy may surprise even the most skeptical of your friends.

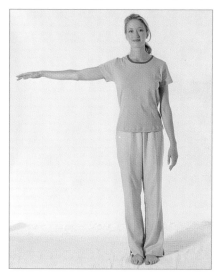

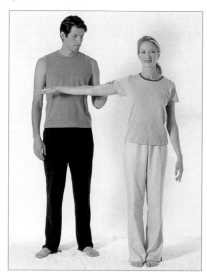

a) Extend your arm to the side and raise it to shoulder height.

b) To test your normal muscle strength, ask your partner to place two fingers on the upper part of your extended arm. Then ask them to press their fingers gently downward while you resist their downward pressure.

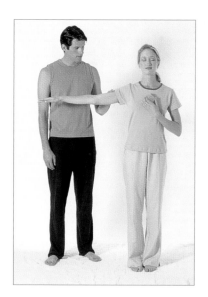

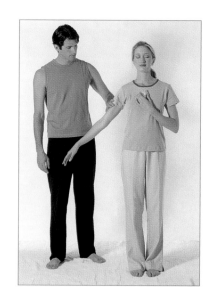

c) Pick up a crystal and hold it over your heart area.

d) Ask an appropriate question, such as "Is this the right crystal for me?" or "Is this crystal good for healing?" or "Is this crystal good for meditation?"

e) After each question, ask your partner to press their fingers gently downward onto your arm while you resist their pressure. If your arm stays strong, this is the "right" crystal for you, but if your arm weakens, try the same test using another crystal.

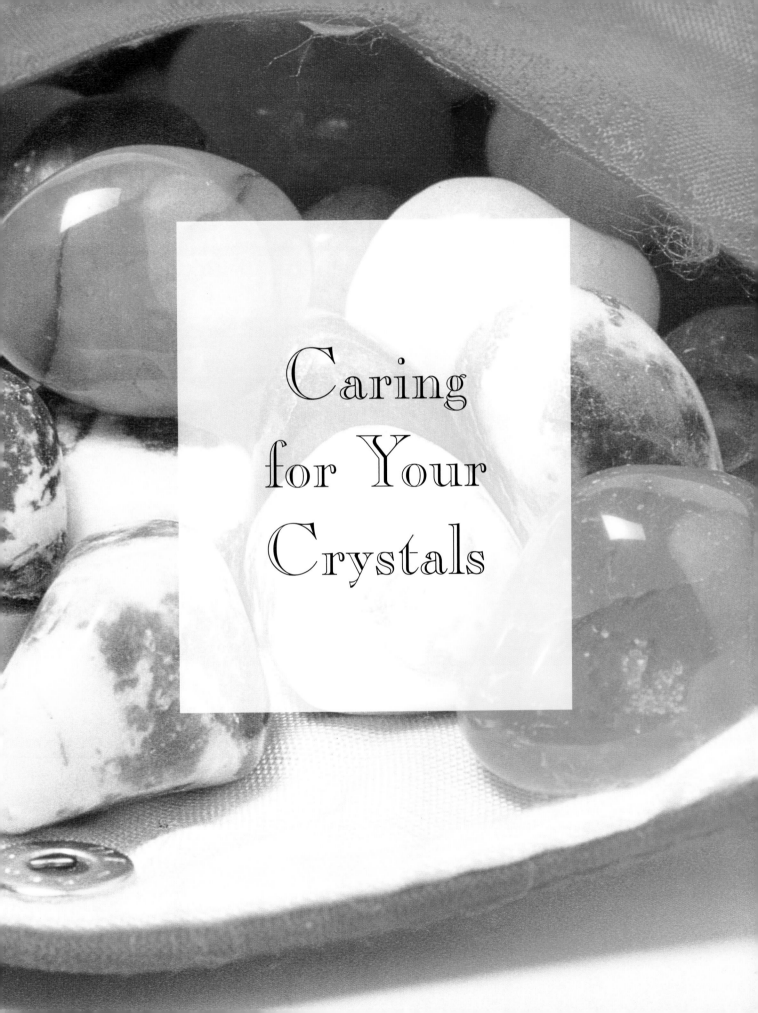

Caring for Your Crystals

Caring for Your Crystals

Being sacred and precious, crystals should always be treated with the utmost care. Although they may feel hard, they can still be scratched, chipped, or even broken. Take extra care when transporting crystals, and always wrap them individually. Tumbled stones are probably the hardiest stones, whereas crystal clusters are the most fragile.

If you intend to carry a crystal around with you, never throw it into your purse or pocket, where it is likely to be scratched or chipped by items like keys or coins. Instead, place each of your treasured crystals singly in a pouch to prevent them from being damaged.

If you wear a crystal necklace, always remove it when taking a bath and take particular care when swimming in the sea or swimming pool. Not only could your crystal suffer damage, but you could lose it altogether if the chain breaks.

Tumbled stones are the most suitable for carrying in your pocket since they are fairly hardy.

Crystal clusters are less durable.

Cleansing Your Crystals

Because crystals can attract and absorb all kinds of vibrations, both positive and negative, it is crucial that you cleanse them to remove any negative energy, both prior to use and on a regular basis. If you purchased your crystals, they will usually have traveled hundreds—even thousands—of miles before reaching the outlet from which you bought them, and will have accumulated within them the energies and imprints of those who mined and transported them. In addition, while they were waiting to be sold they were probably picked up by many more hands and will therefore have absorbed many more vibrations from the individuals with whom they had contact. Remember that negative thoughts, as well as diseases, could have been accumulated by the crystal and may then be passed on to you.

There are many methods of cleansing crystals, and whichever you use is entirely a matter of personal preference. The only thing that you should never do is to use detergents or soap to cleanse your crystals, which would have an adverse effect. All of the following cleansing methods are very successful.

1. Water Cleansing

Water cleansing is particularly suitable for those born under a water sign in the Western zodiac.

A) CLEANSING WITH NATURAL WATER

Take your crystals to a natural source of clean, fresh water, such as the sea, a spring, a stream, or a waterfall, and either place them in the sea or hold them under the running water. (If there is no source of pure water nearby, you can use bottled spring water.)

Never dry your crystals on a towel or a cloth. Instead, allow them to dry naturally, preferably in the sun, which will reenergize them.

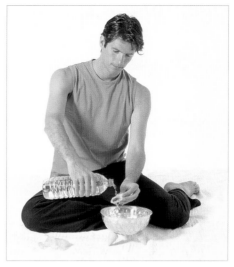

Cleansing with natural water.

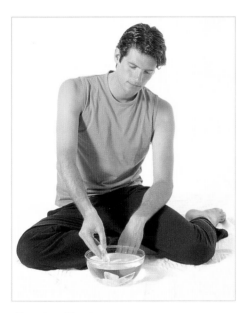

Cleansing with salt water.

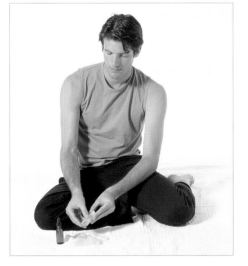

Cleansing with holy water.

B) CLEANSING WITH SALT WATER

Fill a large ceramic or glass bowl with cold or tepid water (do not use hot water, which could cause your crystals to split or fracture). Add a handful of sea salt to the water and immerse your crystals in it for a few hours. Rinse your crystals thoroughly afterward to remove any salt residue and then allow them to dry naturally.

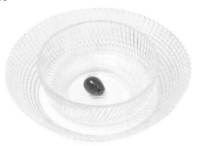

Alternative salt-cleansing method.

Take great care when cleansing your crystals with salt, particularly if the salt comes into direct contact with them. Salt has a chemical reaction with some crystals, causing damage to the crystalline structure, making a crystal lose its polished finish or even causing color changes. If an opal is placed in dry salt, for example, the salt extracts the water from the opal and changes it into chalcedony, a much cheaper stone. However, since using salt is a very effective cleansing method, a safer alternative is to put the crystal in a small glass dish and then to place it in a larger dish full of salt. Even though the stone is not in direct contact with the salt, the cleansing process will still take place.

C) CLEANSING WITH HOLY WATER

You can also rub a few drops of holy water on your crystals to purify them and lift their vibrations. There are many sacred sites around the world where you can collect holy water, including the Chalice Well in Glastonbury, England. Remember to allow your crystals to dry naturally.

2. Earth Cleansing

Earth cleansing is particularly suited to those born under an earth sign in the Western zodiac.

To cleanse your crystal with earth, bury it in your garden and leave it for at least twenty-four hours. Make sure that you remember where you have buried it—it is a good idea to mark the spot—and watch out if you have pets in case they dig it up. If you do not have a garden, or the soil is too acidic (which could damage it), you can bury your crystal in a plant pot. After you have removed your stone from the earth, rinse it thoroughly in pure water and let it dry naturally.

3. Fire Cleansing

Fire cleansing is particularly suitable for those born under fire signs in the Western zodiac.

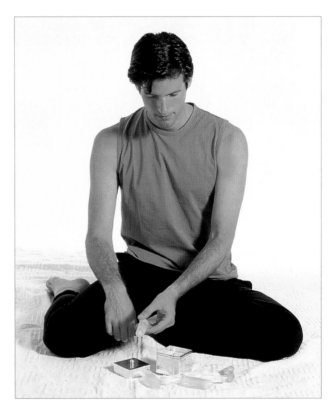

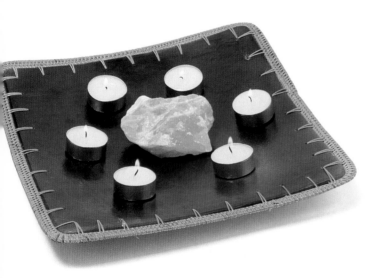

One fire-cleansing method is to surround your crystal with night-lights and then to leave them for several hours until they have burned out.

Alternatively, you could light a candle and very quickly pass your crystal through the flame. Note that if your crystal is an opal, however, the first method is the safest because opals can be damaged by fire.

WARNING: Never leave burning candles unattended.

4. Smudging

The smudging method is particularly suitable for those born under air signs in the Western zodiac.

Smudging is excellent for cleansing, not only crystals, but also rooms and auras. In Native American tradition, smudging plays a very important role. Smudge sticks are tightly bound bundles of plant material. Sage is a particularly purifying herb to include, but cedar, lavender, and sweet grass are also commonly used.

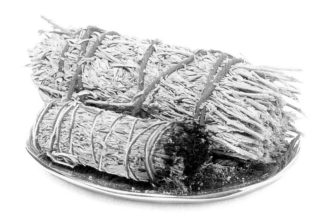

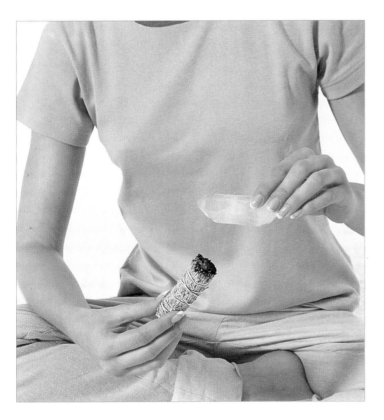

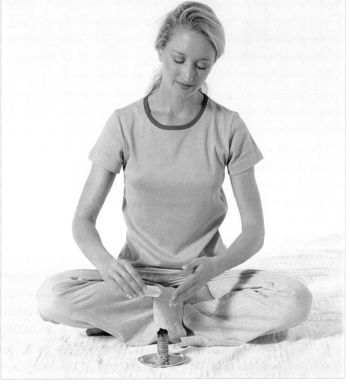

Light your smudge-stick bundle at one end, and, as it catches fire, blow it out so that it is just smoldering. Slowly move your crystal in the smoke so that every facet is treated, thereby allowing the element of air to transmute any negative energy.

If you prefer, you could use a feather or your hand to direct the smoke from the smudge-stick bundle toward your crystal. Make sure that you have a small saucer or bowl to hand to catch any ash and to stub the smudge stick out in.

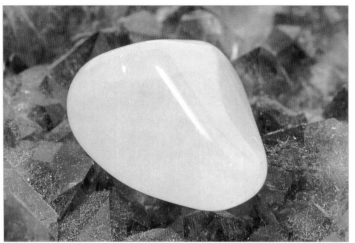

5. Cleansing With a Crystal Cluster

Another excellent cleansing method is to place your crystal on a large, quartz crystal cluster or a bed of amethyst. Leave it there for a few hours to neutralize any negative vibrations.

6. Flower Cleansing

A beautiful and gentle method of purification is to use flowers or petals. Pink rose petals are ideal for cleansing rose quartz, while lavender is wonderful for purifying purple stones, such as amethyst.

Collect some petals and flowers to which you are particularly attracted and place them in a glass container. Now bury your crystal in the petals or flowers and leave it there for approximately twenty-four hours. You could then leave the crystal outside to be bathed in moonlight—particularly if it is a full moon—or to catch the rays of the sun.

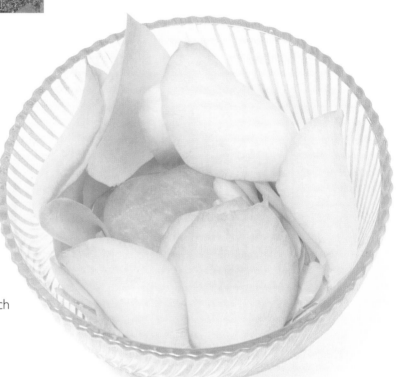

7. Rice Cleansing

To cleanse your crystal using rice, fill a glass bowl with organic, uncooked brown rice and bury the crystal in the rice. Wait for twenty-four hours before removing it, by which time the rice will have absorbed any negative vibrations. The rice should be discarded after use and should not be eaten.

8. Mantra Cleansing

A mantra, such as "Om," may be employed to cleanse your crystals. "Om namah Shivaya" is highly effective for clearing negative energies because you are calling upon the Hindu god Shiva, who is the destroyer or transformer.

   To cleanse your crystal, simply repeat "Om," or your favorite mantra, over it. As you repeat the mantra, visualize the negative energies in your crystal being replaced by pure energies.

9. Essential-oil Cleansing

Although using essential oils is not a well-known method of cleansing crystals, as an aromatherapist it is one that appeals to me. Especially useful essential oils for purification include the versatile lavender, sage, cedarwood, lemongrass, pine, juniper, rosemary, lemon, rosewood, and vetiver.

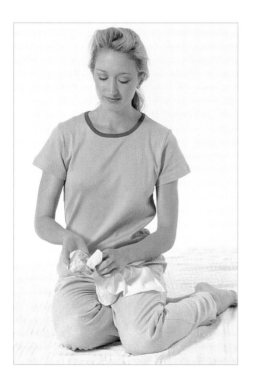
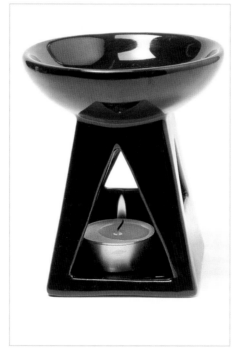
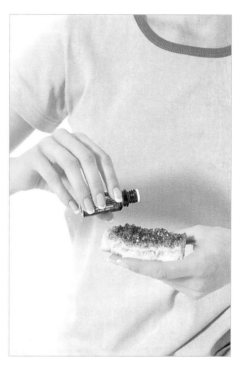

To cleanse your crystals, simply shake one or two drops of essential oil on to a cotton cloth—perhaps a handkerchief—and thoroughly wipe your crystals with it.

Alternatively, you could use an essential-oil burner. To do this, first put a few teaspoons of water into the bowl on top of the diffuser. Then light the night-light underneath the diffuser and sprinkle a few drops of your chosen essential oil on the water. As the vapor begins to rise, hold your crystal in it.

Crystals appear to enhance the aroma of an essential oil. One drop of essential oil placed on a crystal is very powerful and can easily perfume an entire room; the aroma also seems to last for longer.

10. Angelic Cleansing

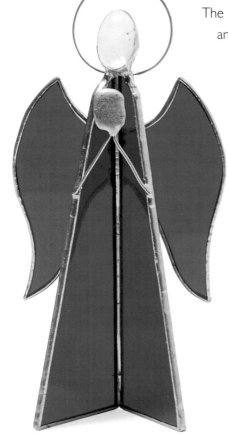

The angelic-cleansing method is not widely known, but it is one that I find both quick and effective. A picture or ornament depicting an angel may help you to focus more clearly.

Place your hands lightly on your crystal and ask the angelic realms to transform any negativity into positive light energy. Calling on the archangel Zadkiel can be highly effective because Zadkiel and the ascended master St. Germain work together with the powerful violet flame of transmutation. Visualize your crystal surrounded by the violet flame of purification.

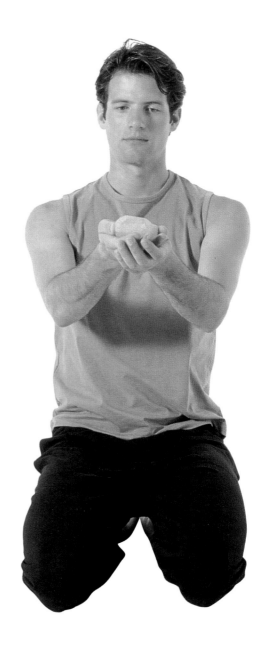

Dedicating Your Crystals

It is important to dedicate your crystal after you have cleansed it because dedication ensures that the crystal will only be used in a positive way for the highest good of all. It also protects the crystal from anyone who may try to abuse its power. Just as crystalline energy can be used for positive purposes, it can also be used for negative ends. Indeed, according to the American psychic Edgar Cayce, the downfall of the lost continent of Atlantis was the result of such a misuse of power.

To dedicate and protect your crystal, hold it in your hands, visualize it surrounded by protective light, and say, "I dedicate this stone to be used for the universal good of all."

Programing Your Crystals

Crystals can be programed for a multitude of purposes, including healing, meditation, and manifestation. The most suitable crystals for programing are clear quartz crystals, which are colorless. (Colored crystals already have their own programs of use—suggested by their color—by virtue of their vibrational and mineral compositions.)

Before programing your quartz crystal, you should be very clear about your intent, which crystals have the ability to magnify.

The following list gives some examples of intent:

❋ self-healing

❋ healing others

❋ absent healing

❋ meditation

❋ angelic contact

❋ protection

❋ harmony

❋ love

❋ the interpretation of dreams

❋ scrying (crystal-gazing)

❋ manifestation

❋ improving your work or home environment

❋ vitality and energy

❋ stress relief, inner peace, and tranquillity

❋ past-life recall

❋ grounding

Once you have decided on your intent, hold your crystal in front of your heart chakra (see page 58) and take a few deep breaths to focus your consciousness and feel the connection.

Then lift the crystal to your third-eye chakra (see page 59) and state your intention clearly, either aloud or nonverbally. Say, for example, "I program this crystal to be used for healing, meditation, manifestation, and communication with the angelic realms." Repeat your intention several times to make your purpose clear.

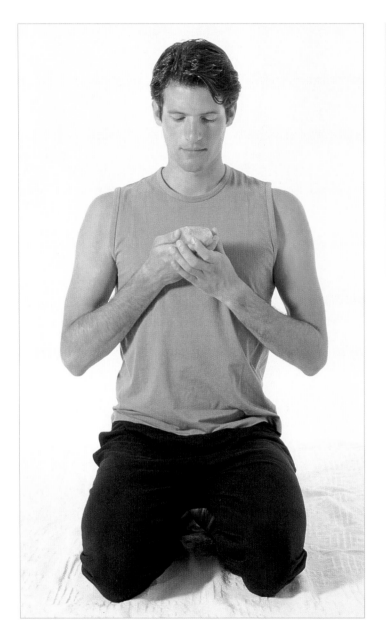

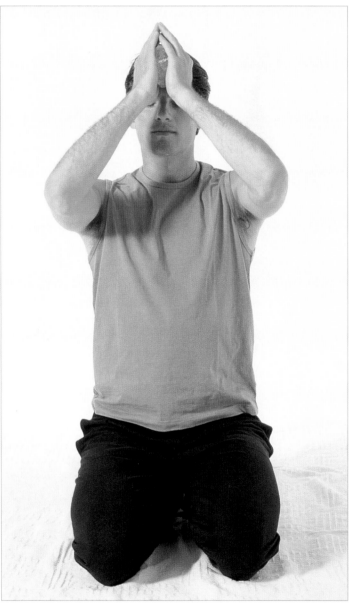

You will intuitively know when the programing is complete. When it is, detach your consciousness from the programed crystal and put it down.

Ways of Using Crystals

Ways of Using Crystals

Now that your crystals have been cleansed, dedicated, and programed, they are ready for use. There is a host of ways in which to use the crystals for healing, and several possibilities are listed below.

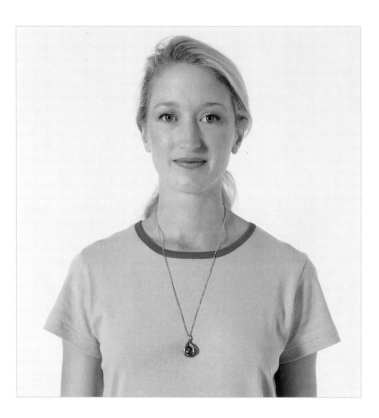

1. Wearing Crystals

Wearing them is one of the most effective ways to use crystals for healing. For best results, the stone should, if possible, come into direct contact with the skin. Women sometimes tuck their crystals inside their bras, while others stick them to their bodies with a plaster. Many people also wear their gemstones in pendants.

The crystal should be worn until there is a positive improvement in the person's health. Although there may occasionally be an initial worsening of the person's symptoms, this is a good sign that indicates that the body's self-healing mechanism has been awakened. This initial deterioration in the person's symptoms is only temporary and should subside within a few hours. If it does not, however, the crystal should be taken off and worn three times a day for about half an hour each time.

2. Carrying Crystals

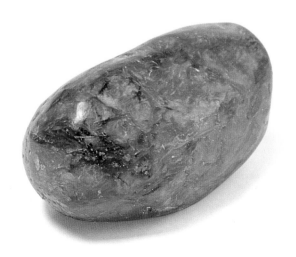

You can also carry your crystal around with you in your pocket (but make sure that you place it in a pouch to prevent it from becoming scratched or chipped). Dip your hand into the pouch from time to time to absorb the crystal's healing energies directly through your skin.

3. Placing Crystals on the Body

Crystals can be placed directly on the body, on a painful area or a diseased organ or joint. They can also be placed on the chakras (see pages 55–66). The stone should be applied very gently to the affected part of the body and then left there until an improvement is noticed. This could take only a few minutes or else you may have to allow fifteen to twenty minutes for the crystalline healing energies to be integrated into the body.

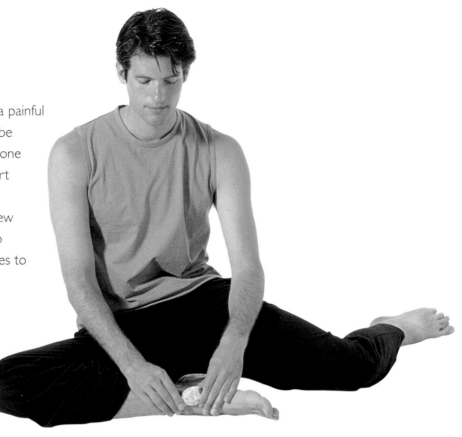

4. Placing Crystals Under Your Pillow

If you place a crystal under your pillow at night, its healing benefits will be imparted to you while you are asleep.

5. Positioning Crystals in a Room

Crystals can enhance your home and working environments. Place them in a position where you can both see them and feel their vibrations, and when you are sitting in their vicinity you should feel physically, mentally, emotionally, and spiritually better.

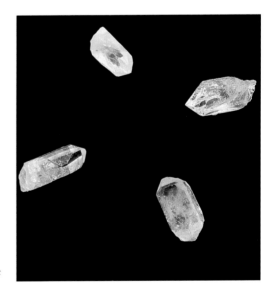

If you wish to promote peace and harmony in your home, place a piece of rose quartz in the room. A piece of purple fluorite positioned by your television or computer will also help to protect you from any electromagnetic emanations.

It is excellent to keep a piece of amethyst or smoky quartz in the work environment because it will absorb any negative energies and protect you from other people's anger and frustrations.

You could also program four quartz crystals for room-balancing and place one in each corner of the room, making sure that each points toward the center of the room. Remember to cleanse your room crystals at least once a week.

6. Meditating With Crystals

Meditation is practiced by many people all over the world to still the mind and achieve inner peace and harmony. Using crystals in meditation will greatly enrich your practice and will enable you to reach higher spiritual levels. Indeed, crystals are the perfect vehicle with which to induce and enhance a meditative state, enabling you to attain a deeper state of peace and tranquillity. Providing as they do the perfect tool to allow you to reach deep within yourself to find your true inner self, at the end of the session you will often have gained new insights, while solutions to problems may have presented themselves, too.

The members of the quartz family are the most popular crystals for meditation, particularly clear quartz, amethyst, rose quartz, and smoky quartz. Different people prefer to use different crystals to enhance their meditation, however, and you should choose the crystals that resonate with you.

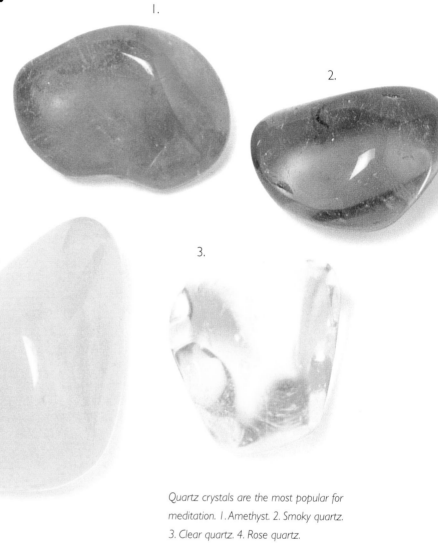

Quartz crystals are the most popular for meditation. 1. Amethyst. 2. Smoky quartz. 3. Clear quartz. 4. Rose quartz.

Before embarking on your journey of self-discovery, consider the numerous benefits of meditation:

✳ it alleviates stress and tension

✳ it lowers blood pressure

✳ it instills a sense of inner peace

✳ it rejuvenates both body and mind

✳ it awakens insights

✳ it accelerates spiritual growth

✳ it clears the mind and improves concentration

✳ it enhances healing abilities

✳ it encourages creativity

✳ it improves health

HOW TO MEDITATE

It is rare for someone to be able to slip quickly and deeply into a meditative state when meditating for the first time, so if you find meditation difficult, do not despair. Be patient—there is so much to discover.

a) Choose a time when you will not be disturbed. Unplug the telephone and tell everyone that you do not want to be interrupted.

b) Make sure that you are not wearing constrictive clothing and surround yourself with pillows for comfort.

c) Wrap a blanket around you in case you become chilly while meditating.

d) Sit comfortably, either on the floor or on a chair. The ideal position is cross-legged on some pillows. It is important to sit upright and to hold your spine straight, helping to establish a strong connection with the earth and enabling your energies to flow freely.

e) Either hold your crystal gently or place it on the floor or on a table in front of you and sit with your hands resting in your lap.

f) Focus your attention on your crystal. Notice its beauty, shape, form, and color. If you are holding it, be aware of its weight and feel yourself absorbing its warmth and energies.

g) Close your eyes and become aware of your breathing. Take a few deep breaths from your abdomen. Inhale for a count of four, hold the breath for a count of two, and exhale for a count of four. Continue breathing in this way until your mind is free from any turbulence. Gently release any thoughts that pop into your head.

h) As you inhale, feel your body overflow with the wondrous healing energies of your crystal. As you exhale, feel the tension in your body dissolving.

i) Allow yourself to sink deeper and deeper into your meditative state. Feel your energy field expanding and filling with beautiful, crystalline energies.

j) Imagine that you are becoming part of your crystal. Allow your energy field to merge with that of the crystal so that you become one with it.

k) If you wish, you could allow yourself to enter your crystal and explore its magical inner kingdom. Alternatively, you could ask your crystal a question. The first impression or thought that occurs to you will be your answer.

l) Remain in your blissful, meditative state for as long as you wish. When you are ready to return, become aware of your body and your contact with the earth. Gently move your fingers and toes and notice your surroundings.

m) Gently open your eyes. If you find it difficult to ground yourself (see below), earth your energies by holding a piece of smoky quartz, black tourmaline, or Boji® stone.

n) Write down your experience straightaway, as spontaneously as you can. Never dismiss as being unimportant any impressions or guidance that you have received while in your meditative state.

THE IMPORTANCE OF GROUNDING

At the end of a meditation, it is vital that you ground, center, and earth yourself. Some people find this much easier than others.

You are not properly grounded if you feel "spacey," detached from reality, or fuzzy-headed. If you experience any of these symptoms, either hold a grounding crystal (such as a smoky quartz, black tourmaline, or another black stone) between your hands, or one crystal in each hand, until you feel more balanced. If you still don't feel fully conscious, sip from a glass of water. To earth yourself totally, go outside and stamp on the ground or even go for a brisk walk. Carrying out boring, mundane tasks like vacuuming or washing the dishes is also an excellent way of bringing you back to reality.

7. Crystal-mandala Meditation

A mandala is a sacred form or pattern that is used as an aid to meditation. It helps to calm the mind and is also wonderful for self-healing. If you are finding it difficult to meditate, the very act of making a crystal mandala will focus your mind and enable you to absorb the energies of your crystals.

To make a mandala, first gather together your stones (tumbled stones, crystal clusters, and long or short crystals are all excellent). Although it is not essential to use every one of them, you should make sure that they have been cleansed before using them.

Sit on the floor and start to arrange your stones. Choose a crystal that you have a particular affinity with as your centerpiece. There are no rules and regulations surrounding the creation of a mandala, so allow yourself to be totally guided by your intuition. Place a piece of material on the floor. Silk, satin, or velvet are all wonderful fabrics, but you can use any material you like. Choose the color of your cloth intuitively.

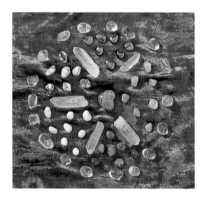

Once your crystal mandala is complete, try the following meditation, either on your own, with a partner, or with a group of friends.

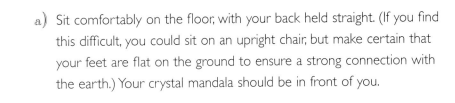

a) Sit comfortably on the floor, with your back held straight. (If you find this difficult, you could sit on an upright chair, but make certain that your feet are flat on the ground to ensure a strong connection with the earth.) Your crystal mandala should be in front of you.

b) Gently focus your eyes on the mandala. Observe the beauty of the pattern that you have created and notice the color and shape of the crystals that you have used.

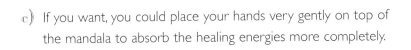

c) If you want, you could place your hands very gently on top of the mandala to absorb the healing energies more completely.

d) Close your eyes and feel the warmth and energies emanating from the crystals. Allow yourself to slip into a meditative state. Remain in this state of peace and tranquillity for as long as you wish.

e) When you are ready to return, gently open your eyes and note how relaxed and tranquil you feel. Make sure that you feel earthed and grounded.

8. Stone-circle Meditation

It is not necessary to go to England's Stonehenge to carry out a stone-circle meditation! This meditation involves arranging stones or crystals in a circle and then meditating within it. You will experience physical, mental, emotional, and spiritual changes as a result of your meditation.

There is no optimum size for a stone circle—it should be whatever size you feel comfortable with. If you feel hemmed in and restricted within your stone circle, then you clearly need to make it bigger. If you are unable to feel energy emanating from your crystals on the other hand, your circle needs to be smaller. As usual, use your intuition when deciding how large it should be. Nor are there any rules and regulations regarding how many crystals you should use or what type. Once again, follow your feelings.

If you are lucky enough to have a room in which you can leave your stone circle, you can spend a few minutes in it whenever you need some peace and regeneration. It is also wonderful to experience this meditation outside, in a peaceful spot on a warm summer's day.

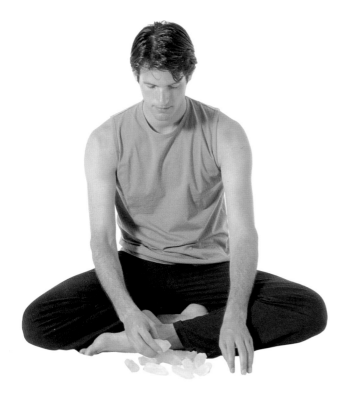

a) Gather together your cleansed crystals. Choose the crystal that is choosing you to hold during the meditation.

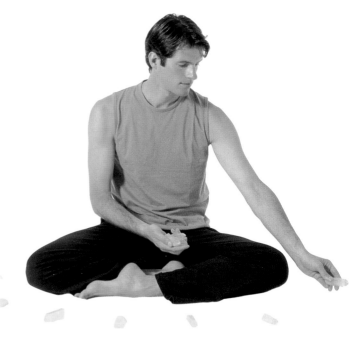

b) Guided by your intuition, start to place your crystals around you. Some people like to use only four healing crystals, arranging them so that they point to the North, South, East, and West. Others like to use seven, nine, or eleven crystals, and sometimes even more. Select as many crystals as you wish.

c) Once you have placed your crystals in a circle around you, settle yourself comfortably. If possible, sit cross-legged in the middle of the circle, but if this position is uncomfortable you can sit on an upright chair (but ensure that your feet are firmly planted on the earth).

d) Gently hold your chosen stone between your hands and take a few deep breaths, breathing in the spirit of love and peace and letting go of your tensions.

e) Close your eyes and feel yourself being totally enclosed by the healing energies of your crystals. Delight in the unconditional love, wisdom, peace, and protection that they are bestowing on you.

f) Remain in your circle until you feel that you have integrated the crystal energy. A few minutes may suffice, but you may equally need twenty to thirty minutes to experience this.

g) When you feel ready to leave your stone circle, make sure that you are thoroughly grounded. (Smoky quartz, black tourmaline, Boji® stones, hematite, obsidian, and black agate are all ideal grounding crystals.)

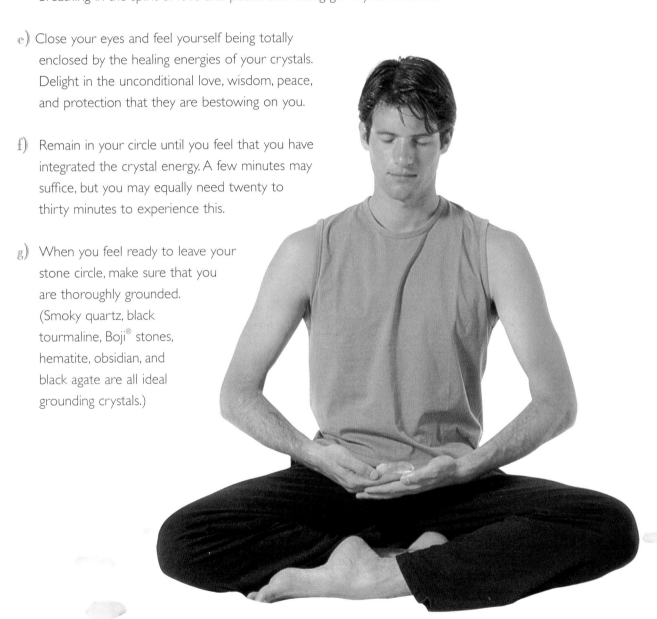

9. Crystal-healing Wands

Being incredibly powerful, crystal wands are among the crystal healer's most potent tools, sending as they do highly focused beams of energy to any area in need of healing. The mystics and healers of countless civilizations have employed healing wands for thousands of years. High priests in ancient Egypt carried wands, and Merlin, the Arthurian magician, also used one. In everyday language we speak to our children of making everything better by waving a magic wand, as does the fairy godmother in the fairy tale and pantomime *Cinderella*.

With a crystal at one or both ends, copper, silver, gold, or platinum wands amplify the energies of the crystal enormously. You can also buy ready-made, "natural" wands that have been cut from practically any type of natural quartz material or gemstone, the most popular including amethyst, smoky quartz, clear quartz, rose quartz, obsidian, and fluorite. (For details of the stones' individual properties, refer to the A to Z chapter, page 67 to page 109.) Alternatively, you could make your own wand.

The wand used in the following treatment was given to me many years ago, when I first started working with crystals. It consists of a hollow copper tube, with a quartz crystal at one end and a copper cap at the other. Some wands have a quartz crystal at both ends. Wands vary in length, but the average size is about 12 inches (30.5 centimeters). Some wand-makers place herbs, oils, crystals, or symbolic images inside the hollow tube before decorating it with metallic threads like those on my wand, although beads and feathers are also often used. If you use a crystal wand like this, you must do so very wisely (when I was first given my wand, I was told in no uncertain terms to use it with the utmost care). For example, when you pick up your wand, be careful at whom you are pointing it and do not leave it lying around.

Rose-quartz wand (above) and amethyst wand (below).

USING A CRYSTAL WAND ON A PARTNER

a) Cleanse and program your wand as you would a crystal to make it ready for use. Have a piece of smoky quartz to hand with which to ground your partner at the end of the session.

b) Make sure that you will not be disturbed during the healing session.

c) Dim the lights or turn them off and light a few candles.

d) Both of you should be wearing loose-fitting, comfortable clothes. Ask your partner to take off any constricting garments, such as neckties and belts, and also to remove any metal objects, like glasses, coins, and keys, from their person because metal produces a false energy field.

e) Prepare a well-padded surface and ask your partner to lie down on their back. Place one pillow under their head and one under their knees to make them more comfortable. This is the best position to encourage relaxation.

f) Position yourself at your partner's head and, using a featherlight touch, either lower your hands on to their shoulders or place them on their head.

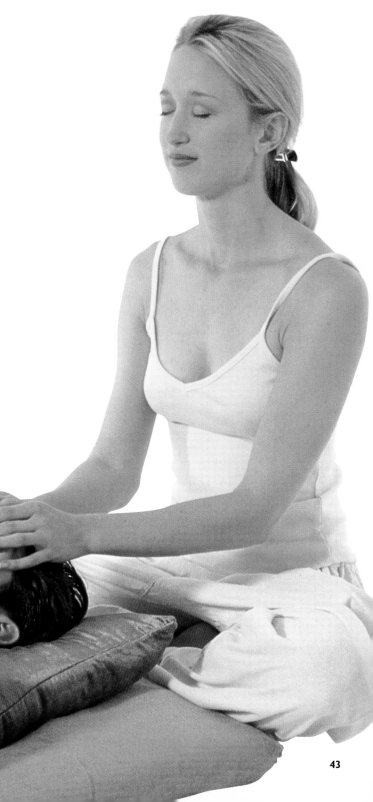

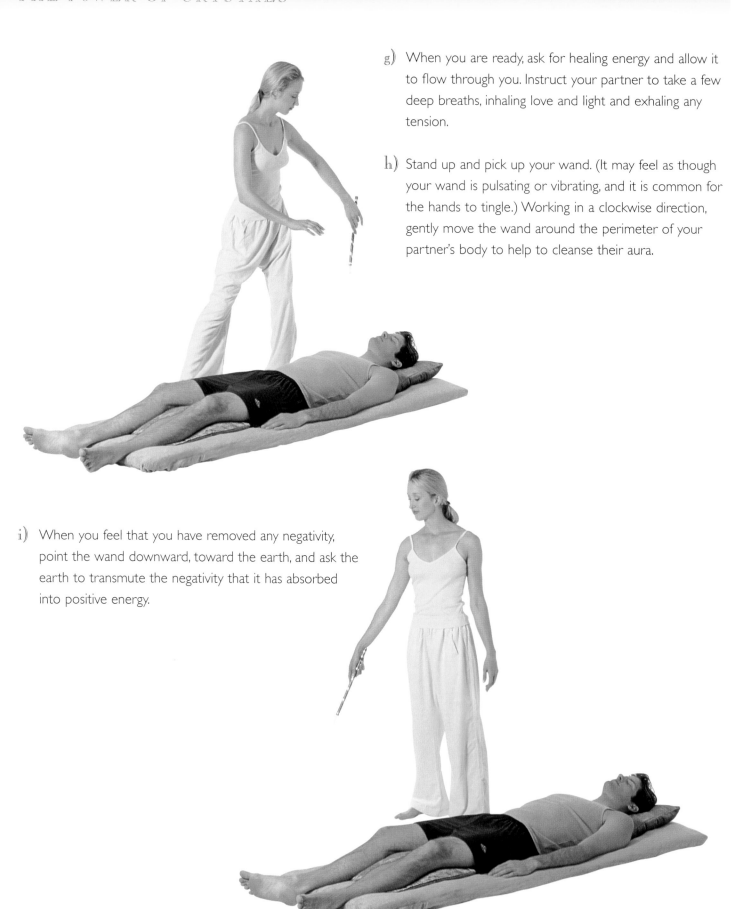

g) When you are ready, ask for healing energy and allow it to flow through you. Instruct your partner to take a few deep breaths, inhaling love and light and exhaling any tension.

h) Stand up and pick up your wand. (It may feel as though your wand is pulsating or vibrating, and it is common for the hands to tingle.) Working in a clockwise direction, gently move the wand around the perimeter of your partner's body to help to cleanse their aura.

i) When you feel that you have removed any negativity, point the wand downward, toward the earth, and ask the earth to transmute the negativity that it has absorbed into positive energy.

k) When your wand's energies feel focused and ready, direct them into the area of your partner's body that needs attention, moving the wand in a clockwise direction. The painful or diseased area will become filled with healing light within a few minutes. Point the wand downward, toward the earth, to transmute any negative energy that has been absorbed by the wand into positive energy.

l) If any other areas of your partner's body require healing, treat them as described in the previous step.

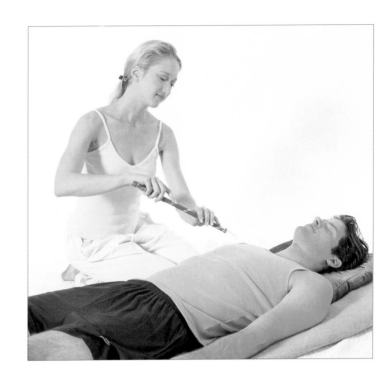

m) Put down your wand in a safe place, ready to be cleansed. Pick up the piece of smoky quartz and place it at your partner's feet to ground and stabilize them. Place your hands on their feet and gently rub their feet and lower legs to ensure that consciousness returns to their body. Ask your partner to open their eyes gently.

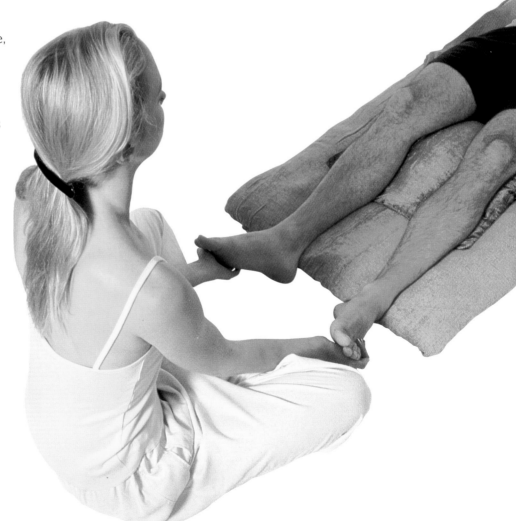

Alternatively, your partner could sit on a chair with their back straight and their feet placed firmly on the ground.

Use your intuition and creativity to find other ways of using your crystal wand. Healing can be directed to difficult situations, troubled areas of the world, or to the earth itself, as well as to people.

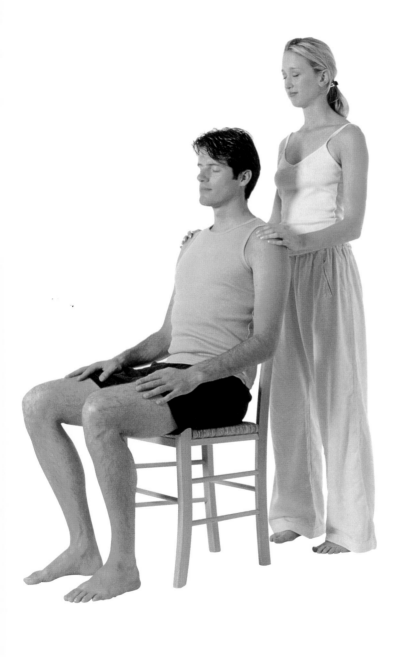
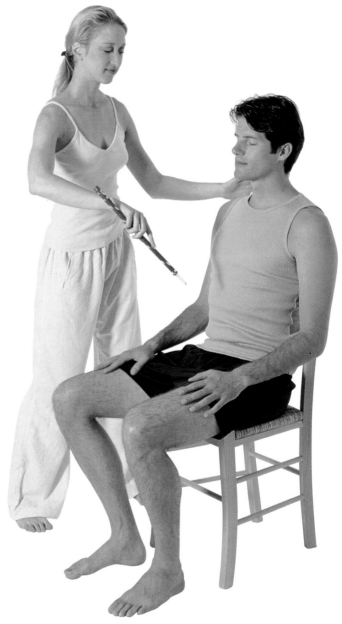

10. Scrying

Scrying is an ancient method of divining, using either crystals or a crystal ball.

CHOOSING A CRYSTAL BALL

Crystal balls are traditionally used to gaze into the past or future or to help one to evaluate a current situation. You can work with a large, clear, quartz crystal, a crystal ball or egg, or even a crystal pyramid. As usual, use your intuition when choosing your crystal.

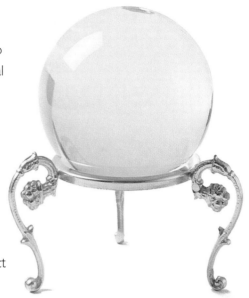

Although most are colorless, which appears to enhance communication, it is possible to buy amethyst, selenite, or obsidian crystal balls. I personally feel that it is easier to scry with a clear crystal ball, but you should be guided by what feels right. Make sure that you pick up several before making your selection. Which size feels right to you? Which one feels most comfortable to hold?

When you have chosen your crystal ball, cleanse it using one of methods described earlier. Charge it on the night of a full moon, store it in a cloth to protect it, and don't let anyone else touch it.

USING A CRYSTAL BALL

a) Spread out a cloth and place your crystal ball on it, resting it on its stand.

b) Dimming the lights and lighting a few candles should make it easier for you to read your crystal ball, but if you feel happier in bright light, this is perfectly acceptable. Settle yourself comfortably, making sure that your crystal ball is easily accessible.

c) Focus on your breathing and take several deep breaths to release any stress and tension.

d) Hold your crystal ball for a while as you begin to focus on a question. Now put it down again.

e) Relax, cup your hands over your crystal ball, and gaze dreamily into it. It may appear to mist over, with pictures or symbols starting to appear out of the mist, or else guiding thoughts may come to you. Don't try too hard or worry if you don't receive an impression immediately. You can always try again tomorrow, so be patient. Gazing into your crystal ball little and often is far more effective than staring into it for an hour.

f) Give thanks to both your higher self and your crystal ball for any communication or guidance that you have been given.

g) Write down any impressions that you received, even if they seem ridiculous: you may be able to make sense of them later on.

h) Make sure that you feel properly grounded.

i) Wrap your crystal ball in its cloth and put it away in a safe place.

Crystal Massage

Not only is giving or receiving a massage a wonderful experience, but this ancient healing art is beneficial to all of the systems of the body. Massage has a powerfully sedative effect on the nervous system, gently soothing away stress and tension; easing muscular aches and pains; improving muscle tone; alleviating stiffness of the joints; improving circulation and the function of the heart; slowing and deepening breathing; eliminating waste products; enhancing digestion and relieving constipation; and alleviating menstrual problems.

Crystals can be used in a treatment to enhance the therapeutic effects of massage. Indeed, some therapists find that patients respond more rapidly when crystals are used in a massage treatment.

Although massage is very safe, there are occasions when it should be avoided, so please note the following contraindications:

* thrombosis—massage could dislodge a blood clot, causing a stroke or heart attack

* severe varicose veins

* infectious diseases, such as scabies, ringworm, and chicken pox

* areas of sepsis (i.e., the presence of pus)

* cuts and wounds

* recent scar tissue

* areas of inflammation

* in pregnancy when there is a history of miscarriage

* fevers

Preparing for a Crystal Massage

Choose a time when you will be undisturbed and take the phone off the hook.

• Try to create the right ambience by playing some relaxation music, dimming the lights, and lighting a few candles. Essential oils will give your room a pleasant aroma, and frankincense, rosewood, cedarwood, jasmine, rose, neroli, sandalwood, and linden blossom all enhance spiritual awareness.

Prepare your massage surface with care.

• Wear comfortable, loose-fitting clothing that will enable you to move around easily. Take off your watch and any other jewelry that may scratch the receiver. Clip your fingernails, too.

• Prepare your massage surface. Although a professional massage therapist will have a couch, this is not essential. You could simply place a thick comforter, sleeping bag, or one or two thick blankets on the floor and have a few pillows and towels to hand.

✳ Select a suitable carrier oil, such as a pure, good-quality vegetable, nut, or seed oil, which should be cold pressed, unrefined and additive-free. *Do not* use a mineral oil like commercial baby oil, which is lacking in nutrients and is not easily absorbed. Sweet-almond, peach-, or apricot-kernel oils are particularly suitable because these carrier oils are neither too thick nor have a strong odor and are also readily absorbed by the skin.

✳ You may add essential oils to your carrier oil, although remember that they must be used with great care and must never be used undiluted. Add three drops of essential oil to two teaspoons (10 milliliters) of carrier oil. The essential oils that help us to become attuned to the spiritual realms include bergamot, clary sage, elemi, frankincense, grapefruit, jasmine, linden blossom, mandarin, myrtle, neroli, rose, and sandalwood. To remove physical, emotional, and spiritual blockages, try cedarwood, frankincense, juniper, rosewood, and yarrow.

✳ Select at least one clear quartz crystal that you have previously cleansed. (You will need two stones to carry out the complete crystal massage as described below.) You will also need a stone for grounding your receiver, such as smoky quartz, hematite, obsidian, black tourmaline, or a Boji® stone. Make sure that your crystals have no sharp, chipped edges that could damage your receiver. Alternatively, you could use a large, tumbled stone or a massage wand. If you want to magnify your crystal massage, you could also select some large quartz crystals to place around the receiver's body.

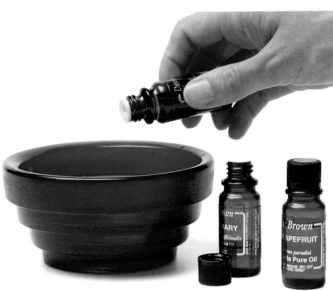

Essential oils may be added to your carrier oil to enhance the effects of the crystal massage.

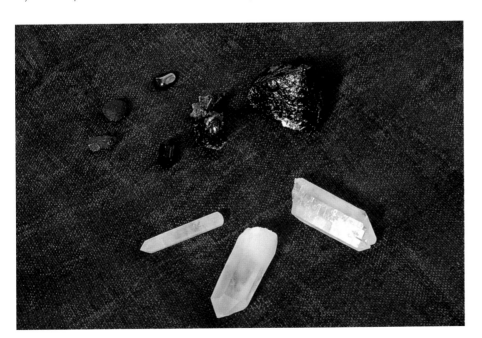

A selection of stones suitable for crystal massage and for grounding the receiver at the end of the treatment.

Crystal-massage Procedure

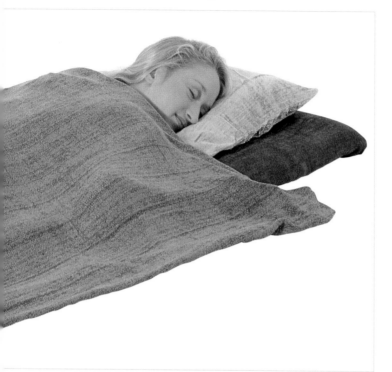

1. Ask the receiver to undress to their underwear and then to lie on their front on the firm, yet well-padded, surface that you have prepared. Place one pillow under their head and another under their feet to make them more comfortable. Cover them with two large towels to keep them warm.

2. (Optional.) If you have selected some large, clear quartz crystals, place them around the receiver roughly the same distance apart, with the points facing inward. Remember to allow enough room for you to enter the circle and give the massage. (You can use as few or as many crystals as you like. I prefer to use between four and twelve, but you, as always, should be guided by your intuition.) When you are inside the crystal circle, you will find the energy emanating from the crystals quite remarkable.

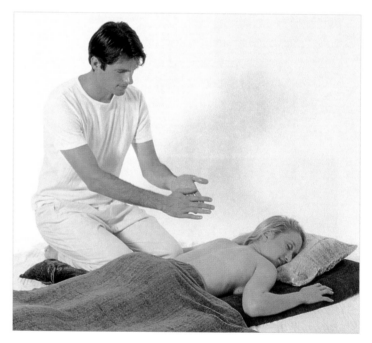

3. Lightly place both of your hands on the receiver's back and feel the tension gently melting away.

4. Draw back the towel and oil the receiver's back, using gentle, stroking movements. Position yourself at the receiver's side, pour a small amount of carrier oil on to the palm of one hand and then rub your hands together to warm the oil.

5. Place the palms of both hands at the base of the receiver's back, one on either side of the spine, with your fingers pointing upward. Now, moving upward (a), and using firm pressure, stroke the receiver's back. As you reach the top of their back (b), stroke outward across the shoulders, using a featherlight touch, and then return to your starting point. Make sure that you mold your hands to the contours of the receiver's body and that you also perform your movements slowly to relax the receiver completely. Repeat as many of these movements as you feel are necessary.

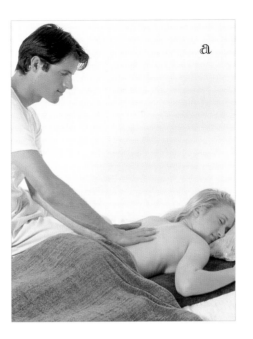
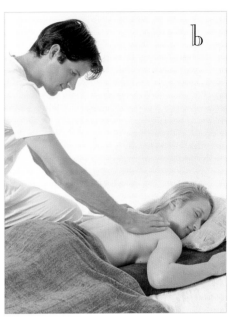

6. Pick up your massage stone or wand and, holding it gently between both of your hands, ask it to balance the receiver's body, mind, and spirit. Using one or both hands, make a large, stroking, circular movement on the right-hand side of the receiver's back and then repeat it seven times.

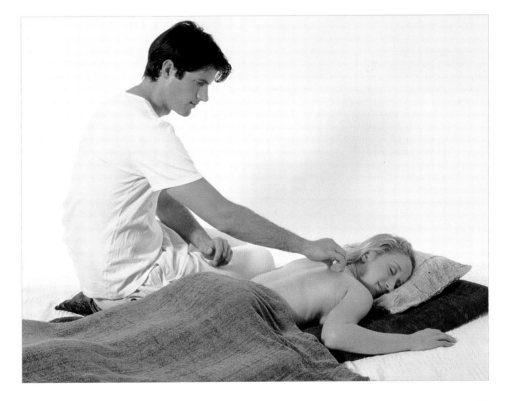

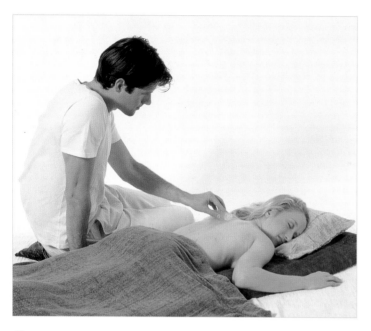

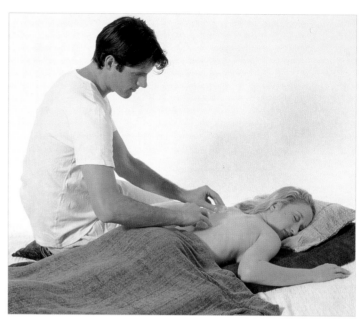

7. Now place your massage stone on the bottom left-hand side of the receiver's back and make a large, stroking movement up it.

8. If you have selected two stones for your massage, place one in each hand and sweep up to the top of the back and down again. Repeat this at least three times.

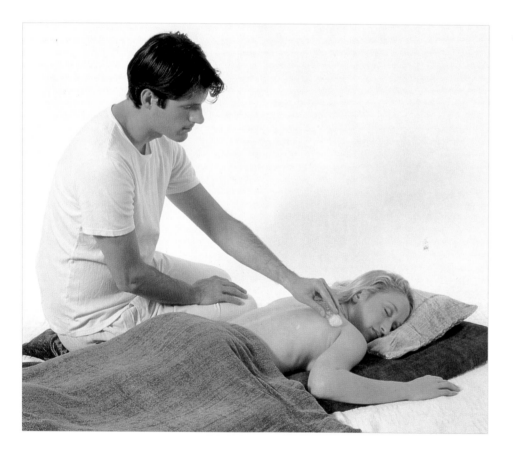

9. If there is a painful area of the body, or an area that otherwise requires attention, pick up a crystal and gently place it over the affected spot. Move it gently over the area in a counterclockwise direction as many times as are necessary to draw out the pain. Gently lift off the crystal and direct any negative energies that may have been released into it at the earth for transmutation.

10. Now pick up the other crystal and gently place it on the area that you have been working on in step 8. Place both of your hands over it and massage in a clockwise direction while asking that the area be filled with healing crystalline power. Repeat steps 9 and 10 on any other troublesome areas.

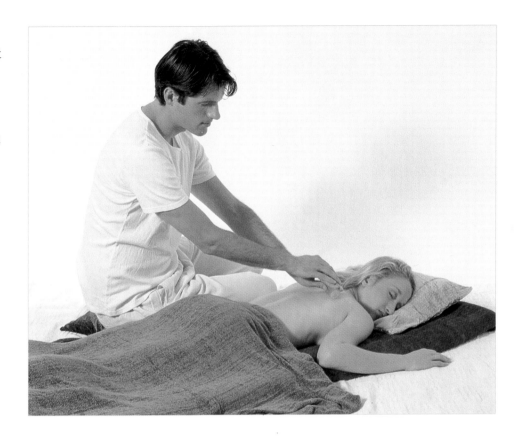

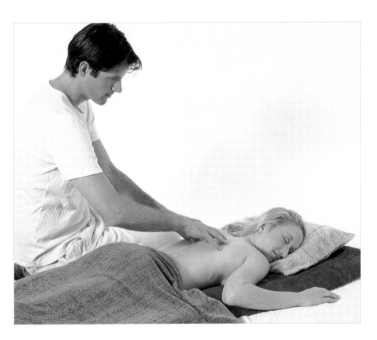

11. Using just your fingertips, gently stroke the receiver's back and then cover it up with the towel.

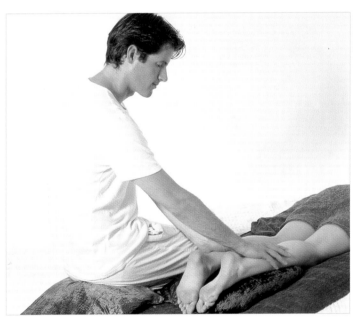

12. Position yourself at the receiver's feet, draw back the towel, and gently place a hand on each of their legs to attune yourself.

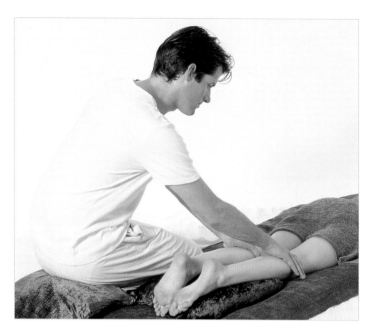

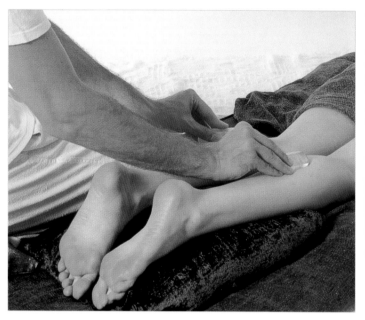

13. Pour a little carrier oil on to the palm of one hand, rub your hands together, and then place a hand on each of the receiver's legs, just above the heel.

   Stroke gently, yet firmly, up each leg, applying hardly any pressure to the back of the knees. When you reach the top of the thighs, allow your hands to glide back to your starting point, using scarcely any pressure. Repeat these stroking movements several times.

14. Now take a stone in each hand and gently stroke up both legs at the same time before gliding back again.

15. Cover up the receiver with a towel and allow them to rest within the healing circle for a few minutes while the crystal energies do their work.

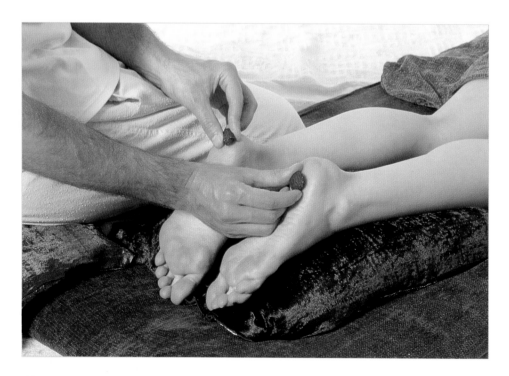

16. Place one or more grounding crystals—perhaps a smoky quartz or black tourmaline—at the receiver's feet. Alternatively, hold a Boji® stone in each hand and place your hands over the receiver's soles to make certain that they are completely earthed.

17. If you have created one, dismantle the stone circle. When the receiver feels ready to come round, offer them a glass of water.

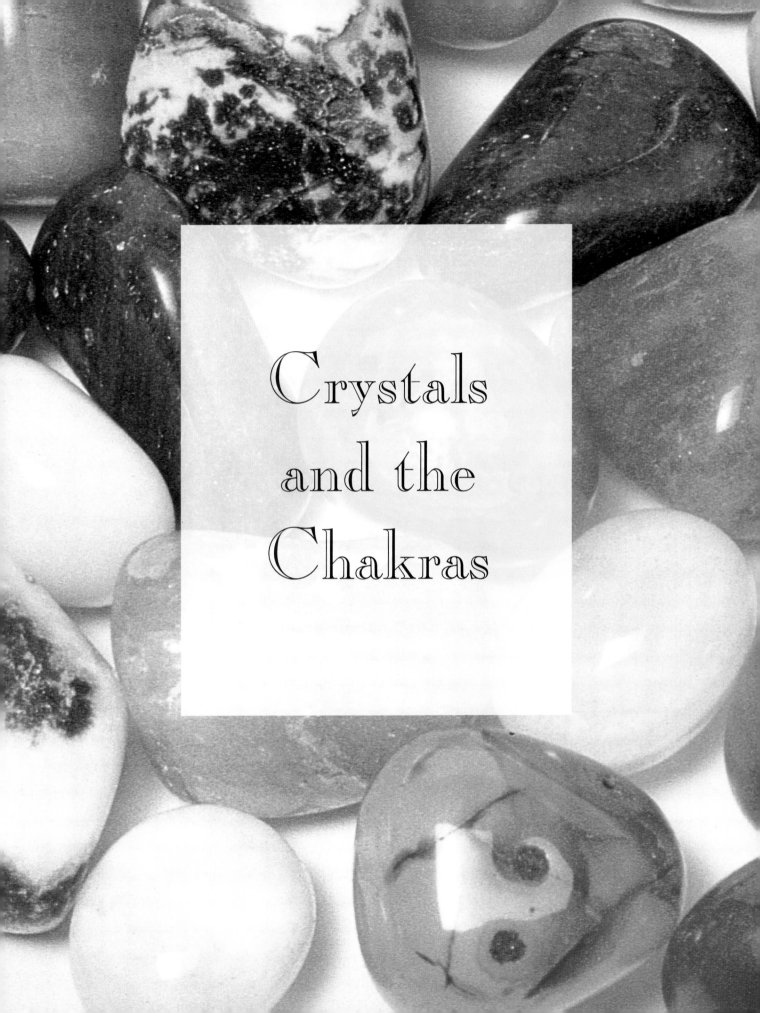

Crystals and the Chakras

Crystals and the Chakras

The word *chakra* comes from the Sanskrit for "wheel," "disk," or "circle." A chakra is like a vortex: a constantly revolving wheel of energy.

Chakras act as bridges linking the physical body with the subtle bodies. If our chakras are not in balance, the free flow of energy, or *prana*, is impeded, leading to physical, emotional, mental, or spiritual unease. When our energy centers are unblocked and free-flowing, however, we enjoy optimum health.

There are many chakras within the body, including the seven major, or "master," ones, which are situated at positions from the base of the spine to the top of the head. I will first describe these chakras before teaching you how to rebalance and align them using crystals.

The Seven Major Chakras

The seven major chakras are:

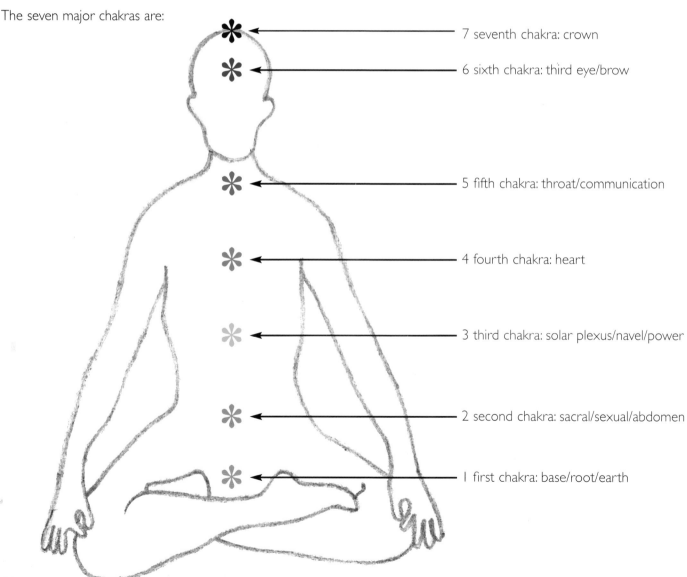

7 seventh chakra: crown

6 sixth chakra: third eye/brow

5 fifth chakra: throat/communication

4 fourth chakra: heart

3 third chakra: solar plexus/navel/power

2 second chakra: sacral/sexual/abdomen

1 first chakra: base/root/earth

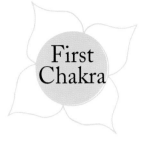

First Chakra

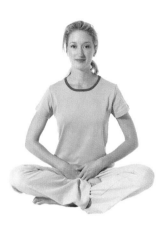

Name: base/root/earth.

Sanskrit name: *Muladhara.*

Meaning: root/support.

Location: base of the spine, in the perineum between the anus and the genitals.

Color: red (representing passion for life) or black (signifying stability or grounding).

Petals: four.

Element: earth.

Sound: *Lam.*

Associated glands: adrenals; some say gonads (i.e., the ovaries or testes).

Associated essential oils: benzoin, patchouli, and vetiver.

Function: the earth chakra is our center of survival and security. If it is imbalanced, we are not grounded or solid and do not have a strong physical will to be on the earth plane. We experience feelings of "spaciness" and have little strength, courage, or stamina. Physical problems relating to the feet, ankles, knees, thighs, lower back, sciatica, bowels, and hemorrhoids are common if this chakra is imbalanced.

Chakra stones: mostly red and black stones, including: fire agate, bloodstone, Boji® stone, red calcite, carnelian, cuprite, garnet, hematite, brecciated jasper, brown jasper, red jasper, obsidian, smoky quartz, ruby, black sapphire, black tourmaline, and zircon.

Second Chakra

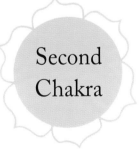

Name: sacral/sexual/abdomen.

Sanskrit name: *Svadhisthana.*

Meaning: seat of vital force/sweetness.

Location: lower abdomen, a few inches below the navel.

Color: orange (representing creativity and wisdom).

Petals: six.

Element: water.

Sound: *Vam.*

Associated glands: gonads (i.e., the ovaries or testes); some say spleen.

Associated essential oils: carrot seed, dill, geranium, hyssop, jasmine, marjoram, neroli, rose, and sandalwood.

Function: the sacral chakra is our sexual, creative chakra. If it is unbalanced, we will have problems forming sexual relationships in particular. An imbalanced sex drive, a loss of libido, promiscuity, frigidity, impotence, or even a sexual perversion may be present, while the reproductive organs may not function effectively, resulting in infertility. Because this chakra is connected with the water element, there may be problems with the kidneys, bladder, or prostate gland.

Chakra stones: mostly orange stones, including: amber, orange calcite, carnelian, citrine, golden labradorite (orange sunstone), tangerine quartz, thulite, and topaz.

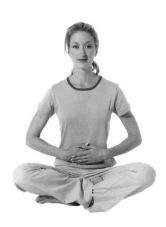

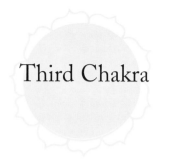

Third Chakra

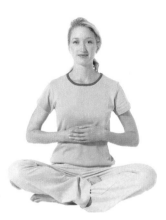

Name: solar plexus/navel/power.

Sanskrit name: *Manipura*.

Meaning: power chakra, lustrous gem.

Location: between the umbilicus (navel) and the solar plexus (representing analytical thought and intellectual activity).

Color: yellow.

Petals: ten.

Element: fire.

Sound: *Ram*.

Associated glands: pancreas; some say adrenals.

Associated essential oils: benzoin, bergamot, chamomile, clary sage, cypress, dill, elemi, fennel, hyssop, juniper, lemon, marjoram, neroli, palmarosa, black pepper, and sage.

Function: the solar-plexus chakra is the source of our personal power, and it is through the solar plexus that we transform our desires, ambitions, and emotions into action. Psychological imbalances in this chakra include a lack of confidence, low self-esteem, emotional instability, addictions, mood swings, and an inability to relax. Physical malfunctions include diabetes, stomach ulcers, eating disorders, such as anorexia and bulimia, allergies, and chronic fatigue.

Chakra stones: mostly yellow stones, including: amber, amblygonite, ametrine, golden beryl, citrine, yellow jasper, smoky quartz, yellow sapphire, sunstone, tiger's eye, and yellow tourmaline.

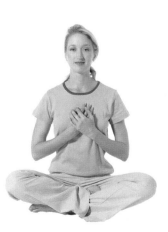

Fourth Chakra

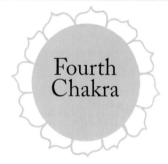

Name: heart.

Sanskrit name: *Anahata*.

Meaning: unstuck.

Location: center of the chest.

Color: green (representing healing and balance) or pink (signifying unconditional love and compassion).

Petals: twelve.

Element: air.

Sound: *Yam*.

Associated glands: thymus.

Associated essential oils: benzoin, bergamot, cinnamon, clove, elemi, geranium, grapefruit, immortelle, lavender, lime, linden blossom, mandarin, neroli, palmarosa, rose, and sandalwood.

Function: the heart chakra is associated with unconditional love and compassion. Imbalances in it lead to an inability to love oneself and others, depression, and difficulties forming relationships. Physical imbalances include circulatory, blood-pressure, and heart problems, asthma and lung diseases, and a poor immune function.

Chakra stones: mostly green and pink, including: amblygonite, green aventurine, green calcite, charoite, chrysoprase, pink danburite, emerald, green or pink fluorite, grossularite, jade, green jasper, kunzite, malachite, moldavite, morganite, peridot, pink petalite, green or rose quartz, rhodochrosite, rhodonite, green sapphire, smithsonite, thulite, pink, green, or watermelon tourmaline, turquoise, and unikite.

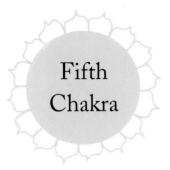

Fifth Chakra

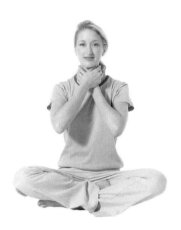

Name: throat/communication.

Sanskrit name: *Visshuda*.

Meaning: purification.

Location: throat.

Color: blue (representing knowledge of, and oneness with, divine guidance).

Petals: sixteen

Element: sound/ether.

Sound: *Ham*.

Associated glands: thyroid.

Associated essential oils: cajeput, blue chamomile, cypress, elemi, eucalyptus, myrrh, palmarosa, black pepper, ravensara, rosemary, sage, and yarrow.

Function: the throat chakra is the center of communication (verbal and nonverbal) and self-expression. Blockages in it lead to an inability to express one's feelings and ideas, throat problems, stuttering, nonstop chattering, or a thyroid or parathyroid imbalance, as well as neck, shoulder, jaw, ear, and hearing problems.

Chakra stones: mostly blue stones, including: blue lace agate, amazonite, amber, angelite, aquamarine, azeztulite, azurite, blue calcite, blue chalcedony, chrysocolla, blue fluorite, lapis lazuli, larimar, malachite, aqua aura quartz, blue sapphire, shattuckite, blue tourmaline, and turquoise.

Sixth Chakra

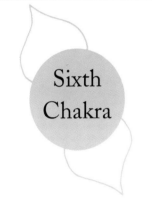

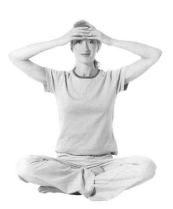

Name: third eye/brow.

Sanskrit name: *Ajna*.

Meaning: to command/know.

Location: center of forehead (representing the search and attainment of spiritual purpose).

Color: indigo.

Petals: two (the two physical eyes surrounding the third eye); some say ninety-six (two multiplied by forty-eight).

Element: light.

Sound: *Om*.

Associated glands: pituitary; some say pineal.

Associated essential oils: angelica seed, basil, carrot seed, clary sage, clove bud, ginger, melissa (true), black pepper, peppermint, pine, rosemary, and rosewood.

Function: it is through the brow chakra that we gain deeper understanding, our intuition is awakened and inner wisdom gained, clarity, vision, and discernment also being developed. Physical imbalances in this chakra include eye disorders, headaches, dizziness, and nightmares. Psychological imbalances include hallucinations, living in a fantasy world, and a lack of imagination and intuition.

Chakra stones: mostly indigo stones, including: amethyst, angelite, azeztulite, azurite, blue calcite, charoite, purple fluorite, iolite, lapis lazuli, larimar, lepidolite, moldavite, phenacite, shattuckite, sugilite, tanzanite, and turquoise.

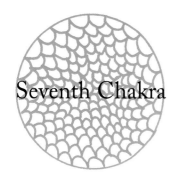

Seventh Chakra

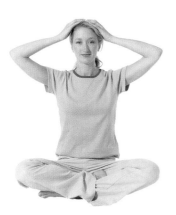

Name: crown.

Sanskrit name: *Sahasrara*.

Meaning: to multiply by a thousandfold.

Location: top of head (anterior fontanelle of newborn babies).

Colors: violet (representing enlightenment) or white (signifying purity, perfection, and bliss).

Petals: one thousand.

Element: thought/knowing.

Sound: silent *Om* or silence.

Associated glands: pineal; some say pituitary.

Associated essential oils: cedarwood, elemi, frankincense, jasmine, linden blossom, neroli, rose, rosewood, and violet leaf.

Function: the crown chakra is our center of spirituality and enlightenment and our link with our higher self. Disturbances in this chakra can cause epilepsy, Alzheimer's disease, Parkinson's disease, memory disorders, obsessiveness, and confusion.

Chakra stones: mostly clear or violet stones, including: amethyst, ametrine, angelite, azeztulite, charoite, danburite, diamond, lepidolite, phenacite, clear quartz, selenite, sugilite, and tanzanite.

Sensing the Chakras With a Partner

Ensure that you are both wearing comfortable clothes, choose a time when you will be undisturbed, and unplug the telephone. To raise the vibrations, light a candle or stick of incense or burn an essential oil.

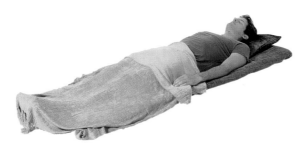

Ask your partner to lie down, on either their front or back, on a comfortable, well-padded surface. Place pillows under their head and knees (you'll also need one to kneel on while sensing the chakras) and cover them with a blanket or towel if you wish. Alternatively, your partner may sit on the floor or on an upright chair, as long as their feet are touching the floor so that they are properly earthed.

You can also explore your own chakras by performing this "sensing" exercise on yourself.

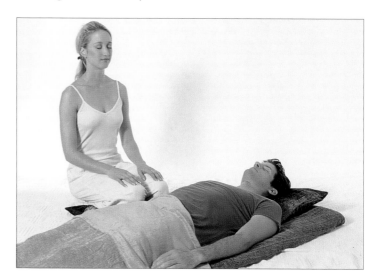

1. Kneel down by your partner's side. Close your eyes and focus on your body and breathing. Ground yourself by visualizing your "roots" penetrating deep into the earth.

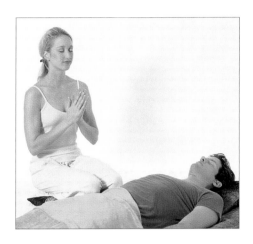

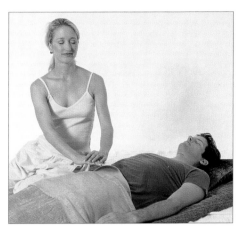

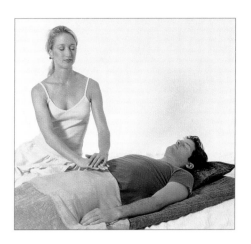

2. Ask your partner to take a few deep breaths and to imagine that they are inhaling healing love and light and exhaling all of their stress and tension. Rub your hands briskly together until your palms feel warm.

3. Gently lower your hands until they are hovering just a few inches above your partner's body, at the base of the spine. This is the root chakra. Try to sense the energy of the chakra as it radiates toward the palms of your hands.

4. Now move your hands up slightly, to the sacral chakra, which is located just below the navel. Feel the energy of this chakra and note what sensation it produces—hot, cold, or tingly, for example.

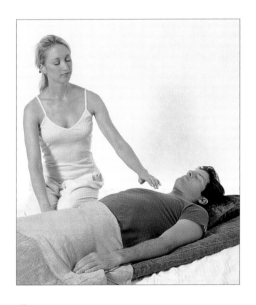

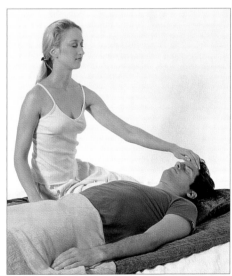

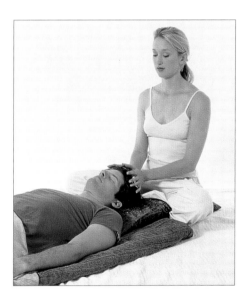

5. Continue your sensing over the solar-plexus chakra (above the navel), the heart chakra (in the center of the chest), the throat chakra (in the throat), and the third-eye chakra (in the center of the forehead), right up to the crown chakra (on the top of the head). Take as much time as you like to complete your exploration of the chakras.

6. When you have sensed all of the energy centers, bring your focus back to your breathing. Place your hands on your partner's feet and gently rub them to ensure that consciousness is within their body. Ask them to open their eyes slowly.

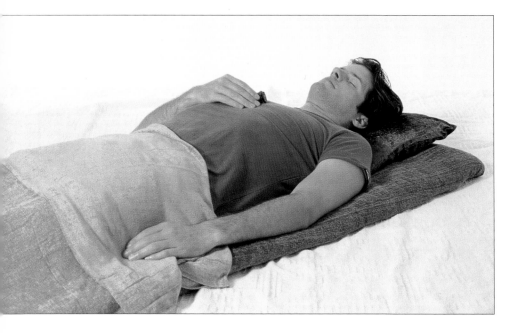

7. Ask your partner to hold a grounding stone, such as a smoky quartz, to ensure that they are completely earthed.

8. Write down any strange sensations that you experienced, as well as any chakras that you felt were out of balance. After you have performed one of the following chakra-balancing treatments, it will be interesting to refer to your notes.

Balancing the Chakras
1. Crystal Layout

Crystals may be placed on the chakras to balance and heal them.

You will need seven stones for a basic chakra layout, one for the color of each chakra. Because you will be placing them on the body, select small ones and make sure that all of them have been thoroughly cleansed. A few suggestions for crystals that would be particularly appropriate for each chakra follow.

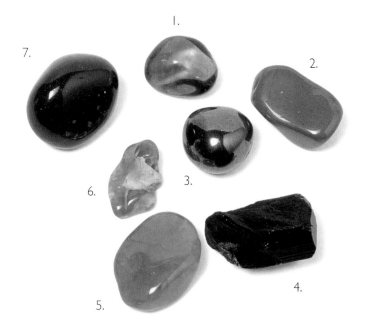

BASE/ROOT/EARTH CHAKRA

Mostly red stones (representing passion for life) and black stones, such as:

(1.) smoky quartz, (2.) red jasper, (3.) hematite, (4.) black tourmaline, (5.) carnelian, (6.) fire agate, (7.) bloodstone.

Also: black agate, black sapphire, brecciated jasper, Boji® stone, cuprite, garnet, obsidian, red calcite, ruby.

SACRAL/SEXUAL/ABDOMEN CHAKRA

Mostly orange stones to promote sensuality and creativity, such as:

(1.) citrine, (2.) topaz, (3.) amber, (4.) thulite, (5.) carnelian, (6.) orange sunstone.

Also: orange calcite, tangerine quartz.

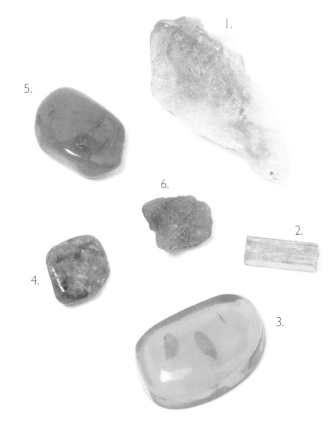

SOLAR-PLEXUS CHAKRA

Mostly yellow stones to release tension, give confidence, and to bring joy, such as:

(1.) amblygonite, (2.) yellow jasper, (3.) amber, (4.) golden labradorite, (5.) tiger's eye.

Also: ametrine, citrine, smoky quartz, topaz, yellow sapphire, yellow tourmaline.

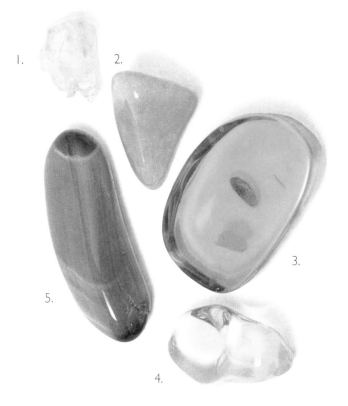

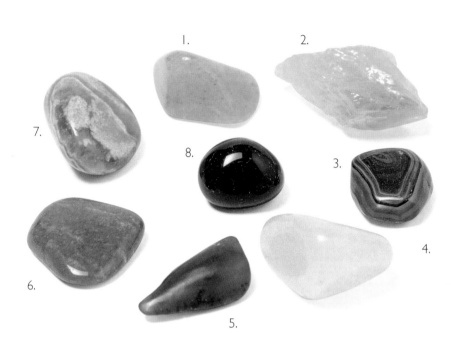

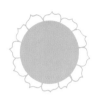

HEART CHAKRA

Mostly pink and green stones to promote unconditional love, compassion, and healing, such as:

(1.) aventurine, (2.) green calcite, (3.) malachite, (4.) rose quartz, (5.) jade, (6.) amazonite, (7.) rhodochrosite, (8.) green jasper.

Also: amblygonite, charoite, chrysoprase, emerald, green or pink fluorite, green quartz, green sapphire, kunzite, moldavite, peridot, pink danburite, rhodonite, unikite.

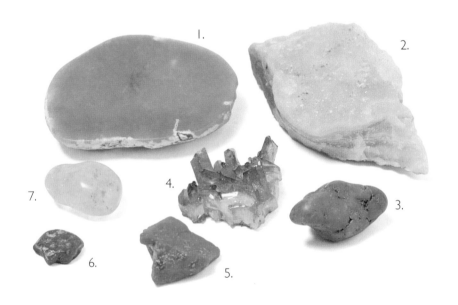

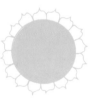

THROAT CHAKRA

Mostly blue stones to encourage communication and expression, such as:

(1.) angelite, (2.) blue lace agate, (3.) turquoise, (4.) aqua aura, (5.) chrysocolla, (6.) shattuckite, (7.) aquamarine.

Also: amazonite, amber, azeztulite, azurite, blue calcite, blue chalcedony, blue fluorite, blue sapphire, lapis lazuli, larimar, malachite.

THIRD-EYE/BROW CHAKRA

Mostly indigo stones to open up the intuition and make us aware of our spiritual purpose, such as:

1.) azurite, (2.) iolite, (3.) tanzanite, (4.) azeztulite, (5.) sugilite, (6.) amethyst, (7.) charoite, (8.) blue calcite.

Also: angelite, purple fluorite, lapis lazuli, larimar, lepidolite, moldavite, phenacite, shattuckite.

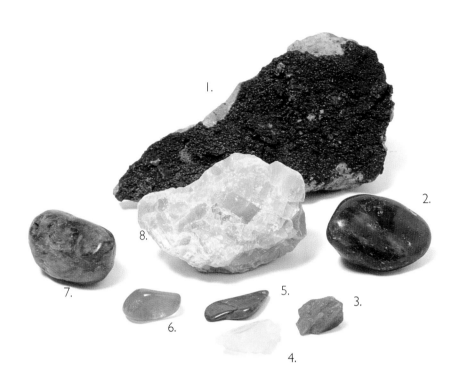

CROWN CHAKRA

Mostly violet and clear stones to connect us with our higher self, such as:

(1.) charoite, (2.) angelite, (3.) clear quartz, (4.) azeztulite, (5.) lepidolite, (6.) amethyst, (7.) danburite.

Also: ametrine, diamond, phenacite, selenite, sugilite, tanzanite.

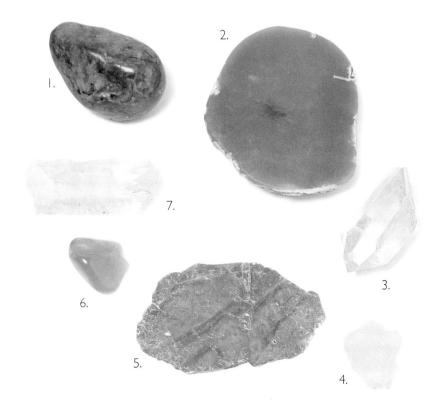

Chakra-balancing Treatment

You may carry out this chakra-balancing treatment on yourself, as well as on a partner. It is not always essential to use seven stones: if you know that a particular chakra needs balancing, then simply place your chosen stone on the chakra that is out of alignment.

If you are working with a partner, carry out the treatment with the receiver lying either on their front or back (whichever is the most comfortable) on a well-padded surface. Place pillows under their head and knees.

1. Having ensured that you are both relaxed, position yourself at the receiver's feet, center yourself, and take a few deep breaths to release any negativity. Slowly and gently place the seven stones that you have selected on each of the

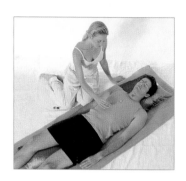

seven master chakras on the receiver's body. Leave the crystals there for fifteen to twenty minutes to enable the crystalline energies to become integrated into the chakras.

2. Remove the crystals very slowly, starting at the crown and working downward. Gently rub the receiver's feet and lower legs to ground and balance them.

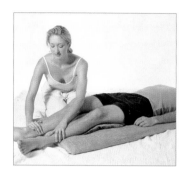

3. When the receiver is ready, ask them to open their eyes gently. Give them a grounding stone if necessary and then offer them a glass of water.

Using a Pendulum

Using a pendulum is another excellent way of balancing chakras. It can also be used for identifying which chakras are out of balance and then aligning them.

1. Ask your partner to lie on their back or front (whichever is the most comfortable).

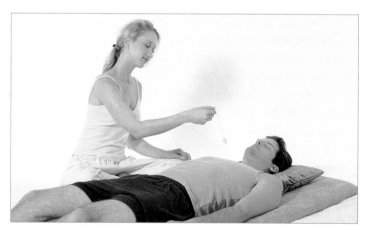

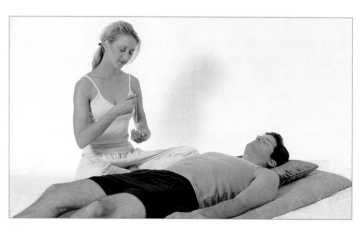

2. Gently hold your pendulum between your index finger and thumb. Do not grasp the chain too tightly in case you prevent the pendulum from moving.

3. Hold the pendulum just above the receiver's body so that it is suspended above the base chakra. Allow it to balance this energy center gently. Although it may move wildly in all sorts of directions as it restores harmony to the chakra, let it complete its work. Continue to work on each chakra in the same way.

4. Once you have completed your treatment, ground the receiver by holding their feet, asking them to hold an earthing stone, and offering them a glass of water.

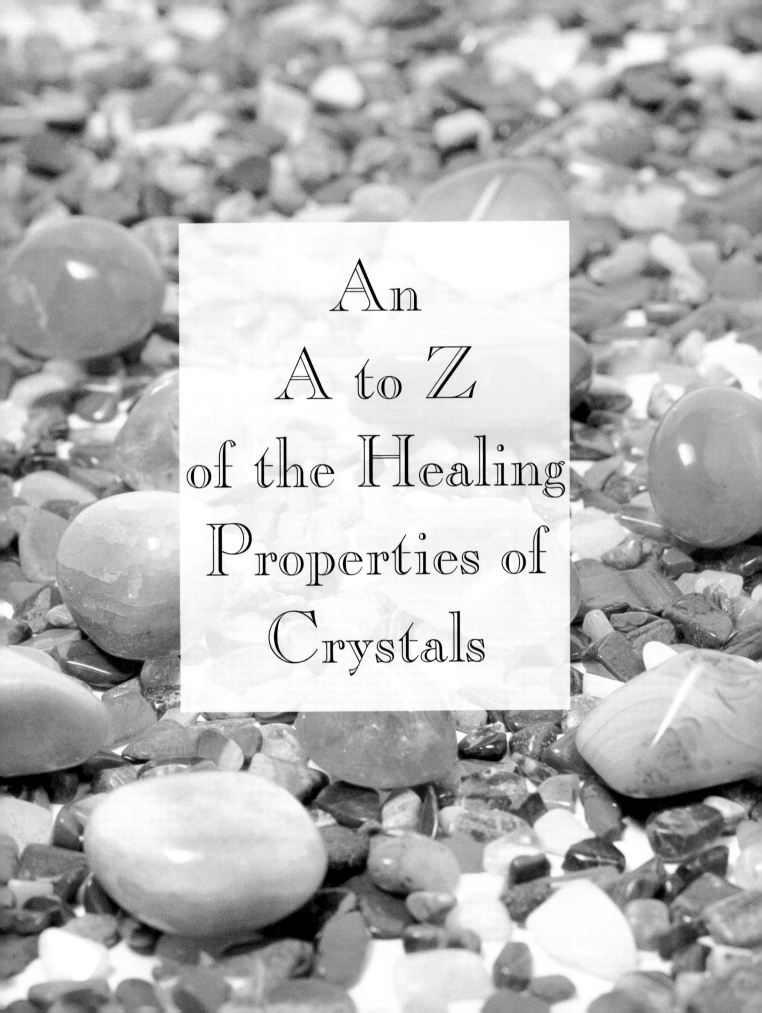

An
A to Z
of the Healing
Properties of
Crystals

AN A TO Z OF THE HEALING PROPERTIES OF CRYSTALS

In this section I have outlined some of the crystals that are most commonly used for therapy. (Although this is not intended to be an exhaustive list, the crystals contained within these pages will give you an excellent introduction.) Photographs accompany each stone as an aid to identification, and if you are immediately attracted to a photograph of a crystal, it is highly likely that you need it, so read the description to discover why. Crystal healing (which is sometimes referred to as crystal, or gem, therapy) is the use of crystals and stones for therapeutic and healing purposes.

Agate

A typical agate usually has a banded appearance due to the deposition of other substances within its layers. Agate is available in a wide variety of colors, including blue, white, gray, brown, red, green, yellow, black, and rose.

In India, Nepal, and Tibet, where agate amulets were popular, it was thought to bring protection and good fortune. Agate is believed to have been one of the stones used in the breastplate of the Jewish high priest in Old Testament times. It was traditionally placed in cooking and drinking water to heal sickness.

HEALING PROPERTIES

Agate is an excellent stone for rebalancing and harmonizing body, mind, and spirit. It also cleanses and stabilizes the aura, banishing negativity.

Agate stimulates and strengthens our analytical capabilities, encouraging us to think clearly and rationally and enabling us to concentrate upon the task in hand. In addition, it allows us to gain access to, and derive inspiration from, the spiritual worlds.

Agate is a wonderful stone to use during pregnancy because it soothes, calms, and balances both mother and baby throughout pregnancy and labor. After the delivery, agate helps to prevent the uterus from prolapsing.

THE HEALING PROPERTIES OF SPECIFIC TYPES OF AGATE

As well as the properties mentioned above, specific types of agate possess other properties.

Blue Lace Agate

Blue lace agate is particularly beneficial for balancing the throat chakra, but also harmonizes the heart, third-eye, and crown chakras.

It is a very calming stone for the mind, endowing us with a sense of peace and tranquillity that enables us to reach an elevated state of spiritual awareness.

Blue lace agate furthermore helps to strengthen and accelerate the repair of bones, as well as cooling arthritic inflammation. It soothes red, sore eyes and any skin problems associated with redness and irritation.

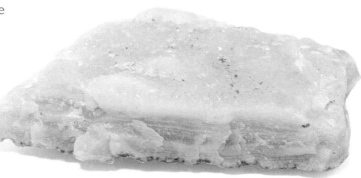

Fire Agate

With its affinity for the base chakra, fire agate is useful for grounding and establishing a powerful connection with the earth. This crystal is excellent for dispelling fear and may be worn to provide a strong shield of protection.

Fire agate may also be used to "burn," destroy, and transmute the old, making way for the new. If there are any aspects of your personality or life that you would like to change radically, this is the stone that you need to "burn" away any blockages or obstacles that are standing in your way. It is also an energizing stone that should be used when you are feeling exhausted and "burned out."

THE POWER OF CRYSTALS

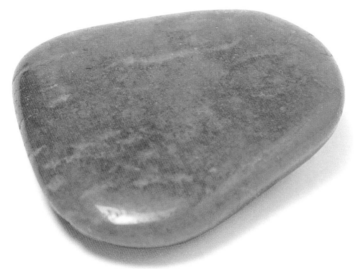

Amazonite

Of a beautiful, turquoise, blue-green color, amazonite is often found with white or gray sections.

According to the Old Testament, amazonite was used in the breastplate of the Jewish high priest.

HEALING PROPERTIES

Amazonite heals the throat chakra, encouraging communication and supporting the thyroid and parathyroid. In addition, it helps to balance the metabolism and regulates calcium deficiencies, also alleviating cramps and muscular spasms.

Amazonite is a wonderful crystal for soothing and harmonizing the nervous system, dispelling worries, fears, anger, and irritation, and balancing mood swings.

It is a stone that encourages us to take charge of our own lives, reminding us that we have the ability to change any situation and connecting us with our own inner power.

Amber

Amber is a transparent or translucent fossilized tree resin that is usually golden or brown in color. Perfectly preserved insects can sometimes be seen trapped within the fossilized resin, providing a glimpse of ages past. If you rub amber, you may feel an electrical charge.

One of the most precious of all "crystals," amber has been used for healing purposes for thousands of years, often as a remedy with a similar effect to penicillin. The Old Testament states that it was one of the gems that was incorporated into the breastplate of the Jewish high priest.

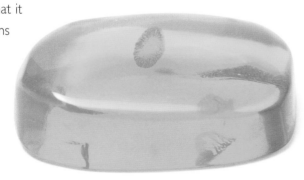

HEALING PROPERTIES

Amber has an affinity for the solar-plexus and throat chakras and may also be used to treat the kidneys and bladder.

A "stone" of purification, amber cleanses the body, mind, and spirit, as well as the aura and the environment. This "crystal" draws disease out of the body, healing and renewing the nervous system and balancing the right and left parts of the brain.

Amber bestows joy and spontaneity, also increasing confidence and, some say, bringing good luck.

Finally, amber possesses timeless wisdom and acts as a record-keeper of the earth, awakening memories within us.

70

Amblygonite

A rare mineral, amblygonite is very light yellow, pink, or lilac and often appears to be white.

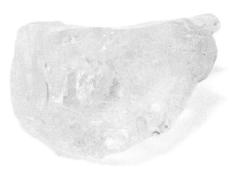

HEALING PROPERTIES

Amblygonite has an affinity for the solar-plexus chakra, as well as the heart chakra. A calming and soothing stone, it helps to relieve anger, irritation, and agitation, instead filling the solar plexus with peace and contentment.

HEALING PROPERTIES

Amethyst has an affinity for the brow and crown chakras and the ability to activate spiritual awareness and psychic abilities. It is a favorite stone for meditation because it encourages one to calm one's mind and fall into a deep, meditative state in which one may discover one's inner wisdom. Indeed, it can be said to bring us that peace that passeth all understanding.

As a stone of tranquillity and contentment, amethyst is excellent for relieving stress and strain, soothing anger and irritability, balancing mood swings, dispelling fear, and dissolving negativity. Additionally a stone of protection, amethyst may be worn to avert psychic attacks and to protect the wearer from all types of harm. With its ability to clear negative and blocked energy, an amethyst cluster provides a valuable addition to any room.

Through its traditional use for encouraging sobriety, amethyst is helpful for those who are trying to give up alcohol, drugs, or other addictions. It may also be used to treat problems of the skeletal system, for reducing swellings and bruises, and for alleviating respiratory, digestive, and skin problems, along with disorders of the heart and circulation, hearing, and teeth. It is frequently used to treat tension headaches by drawing out the pain from the head and may also be placed under the pillow to relieve insomnia.

Overall, amethyst balances many of our physical, mental, emotional, and spiritual aspects.

Amethyst

A highly prized crystal that everyone would benefit from possessing, amethyst ranges from the palest of mauves to deep purple in color.

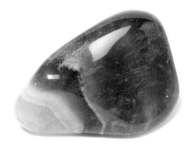

The stone's name is thought to be derived from the Greek word *amethustos*, which means "noninebriated," echoing the belief that it prevented the wearer from becoming intoxicated. It was one of the stones that was used in the breastplate of the Jewish high priest, according to the Old Testament.

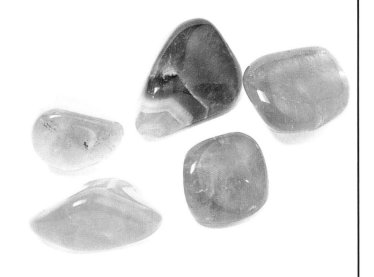

HEALING PROPERTIES

Because it contains purple and yellow, ametrine has an affinity for both the crown and solar-plexus chakras. As an aid to meditation, ametrine enables one to connect with one's spirituality, also opening up one's intuition and bringing forth inspiration and creativity.

Ametrine balances and soothes the emotions, too, bringing peace to a troubled soul by dissolving emotional blockages and transmuting negativity. A dispeller of fears and phobias, ametrine is an uplifting stone that is marvelous for relieving depression and bringing joy to the wearer.

Ametrine is a stone that both instigates change and eases transition, making it useful during puberty or when changes of partner, job, or home are being experienced. Further problems that ametrine has the power to alleviate include allergies, physical, mental, and emotional exhaustion (even M.E.), and digestive disorders.

Ametrine

An unusual stone, ametrine is a mixture of the purple amethyst and yellow citrine and is therefore endowed with the healing properties of both.

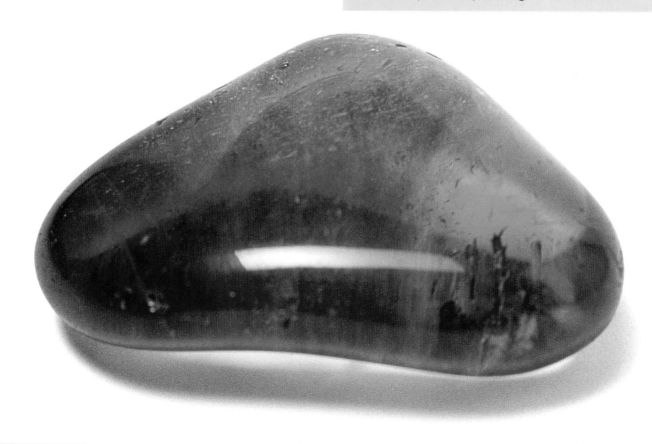

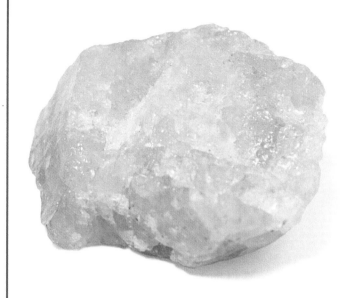

Aquamarine

The name of this crystal is the Latin word for "seawater," a name that reflects its color, which ranges from bluish-green to blue.

Aquamarine was traditionally thought to protect sailors and was said to be the treasure of the mermaids.

HEALING PROPERTIES

Aquamarine is an excellent stone for stimulating, activating, and cleansing the throat chakra. A crystal that encourages us to speak the truth and express our emotions, it also endows us with courage, enabling us to face up to situations and to stand our ground.

Aquamarine furthermore allows us to heighten our spiritual awareness and is useful as an aid to meditation because of its ability to calm the mind while increasing mental clarity.

A beneficial stone for both boosting the immune system and alleviating any over-reactions, such as allergies and hayfever, it may be worn or placed over sore, tired eyes or swollen glands. Because it is a calming stone that eases stress and tension, aquamarine is a marvelous aid to those who clench their teeth and jaws tightly due to anger and frustration.

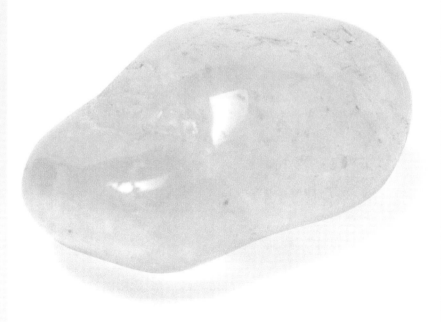

HEALING PROPERTIES

Aventurine is particularly indicated for the heart chakra, which it may activate, clear, and protect, and is generally useful for treating heart problems on account of its ability to strengthen and stabilize the heart, as well as to encourage regeneration.

A stone of comfort and balance, aventurine is favored by healers who wish to promote harmony and wholeness. It encourages feelings of deep relaxation and contentment, filling the heart with love and joy, and is therefore excellent for those who feel unloved or who find it difficult to open up their hearts, to trust, and to form relationships with others.

The physical problems that aventurine can help to alleviate include lung and throat disorders, insomnia, allergies, and skin diseases. It can also provide pain relief.

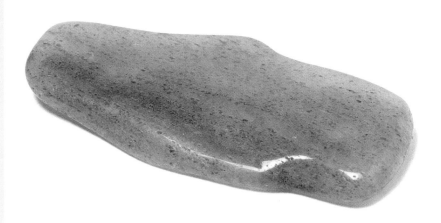

Aventurine

Aventurine's name is derived from the Italian for "chance" or "random," which some say is due to its chance discovery, whereas others say that it refers to the randomly deposited mica particles within it. The color of aventurine is variable, ranging from blue, blue-green, brownish-red, and gray to yellow. The most common color, however, is green.

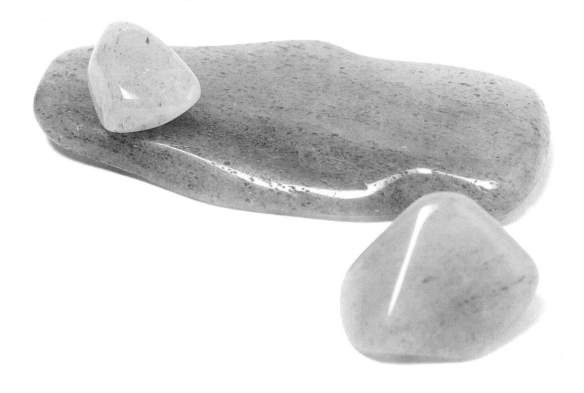

Azeztulite

Azeztulite is a colorless stone that has only recently started to be used in crystal therapy. It is said that azeztulite *never* needs to be cleansed or energized.

HEALING PROPERTIES

With its very powerful vibration, azeztulite has an affinity for the crown chakra. A stone of ascension, it greatly accelerates one's journey toward enlightenment. It may also be used on the third-eye chakra to promote clairvoyance, and, because it brings visions from both the past and the future, is an excellent stone to use when scrying.

This remarkable crystal has been used to treat inflammatory disorders and cancer.

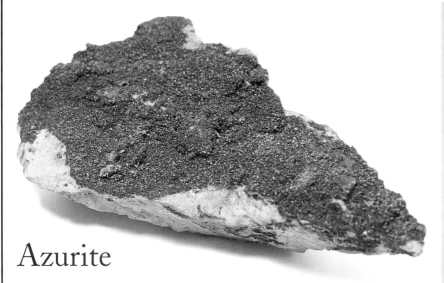

Azurite

The color of azurite ranges from light blue to a stunning deep blue.

Azurite was regarded as a sacred stone by the Native Americans, who believed that it facilitated contact with their spirit guides. The Mayans used azurite to heighten their psychic powers, as well as to transfer knowledge and wisdom via the medium of thought.

HEALING PROPERTIES

Azurite is particularly beneficial for the throat chakra and for activating the third-eye/brow chakra.

Often called the stone of heaven, azurite enables us to receive divine guidance through our higher chakras and bestows the power to develop psychic ability, intuition, and insight.

Azurite has a calming effect on an agitated mind and provides an effective tool for meditation, encouraging us to release our fear and to overcome obstacles that are impeding our progress.

Ailments that azurite can help include spinal disorders and circulatory complaints, as well as liver, gallbladder, thyroid, and throat problems.

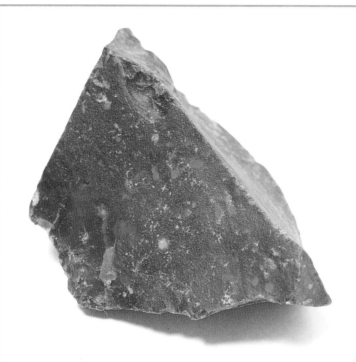

HEALING PROPERTIES

Bloodstone has an affinity for the base chakra, providing solid support and stability. A stone of strength and courage, it is excellent for reinforcing our will to be on the physical plane and to exist in the here and now.

Bloodstone is also useful for alleviating both physical and emotional problems associated with the heart, making it an essential crystal for those who experience difficulties in establishing strong and stable relationships.

Traditionally used to treat blood disorders, it purifies and fortifies the blood, making it ideal for anemia. One of the most effective of all stones for boosting the immune system, it should be placed on the thymus gland, above the heart. Because it reduces pus formation, neutralizes toxins, and stimulates the lymphatic system, bloodstone is highly recommended for healing inflammations and infections.

Bloodstone (or Heliotrope)

Bloodstone is a variety of chalcedony and its color is bright to dark green, spotted with flecks of red (the red spots do not always appear in smaller pieces).

Its alternative name, heliotrope, comes from the Greek word for "solstice," indicating its healing abilities. It is sometimes also referred to as green jasper or blood jasper.

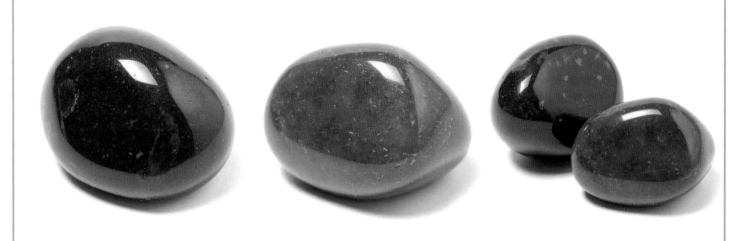

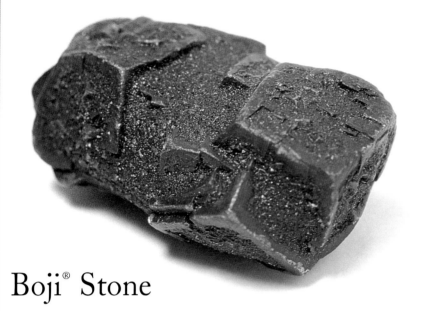

Boji® Stone

Boji® stone is a registered trademark. Although Boji® stones have been around for millions of years, their value and purpose came to light only when they were shown to three-year-old Karen Gillespie by her grandfather. She named the stone after her pet crow!

Brown to blackish stones, usually with a spherical shape, some—mostly smooth—Boji® stones are referred to as female, whereas uneven, bumpy stones with plateletlike protrusions are said to have male energy. A few are described as being androgynous.

HEALING PROPERTIES

Boji® stones have an affinity for the base chakra; when used for grounding, they are excellent for dispelling feelings of "spaciness" because they have a remarkable balancing ability. It is recommended that you hold a pair of Bojis® (one male, one female) in each hand for ten to twenty minutes to stimulate the acupuncture meridians and dissolve physical and emotional blockages. (People often report feeling a mild electrical charge as energy blockages are removed.) Alternatively, you could lie down and position one above your head and one below your feet. They can furthermore be placed on a troublesome area of the body to alleviate pain.

If you carry them around with you, Boji® stones will provide a continuous balancing of energy that also cleans and charges your aura.

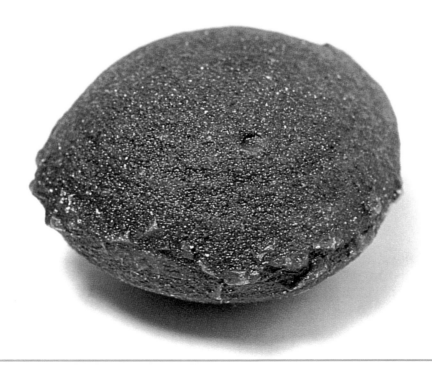

Calcite

Found in a variety of colors, including blue, green, orange, pink, red, and black, calcite can also be colorless.

Calcite (whose name is derived from the Greek word *chaix*, meaning "lime") has been used for thousands of years for healing purposes.

THE HEALING PROPERTIES OF SPECIFIC TYPES OF CALCITE

Calcite is often placed on the corresponding chakra color to clear and activate. I will discuss the colors individually.

Blue Calcite

This stone has an affinity with the throat chakra, its gentle, healing properties soothing inflammations of the throat, as well as treating lung and thyroid disorders.

An excellent stone for reducing stress, anxiety, and negativity, blue calcite also helps to regulate blood pressure. Finally, blue calcite can be used as an aid to channeling.

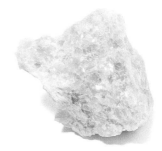

Green Calcite

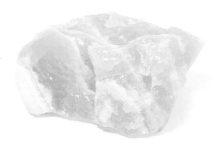

Green calcite is beneficial to the heart chakra and nervous system and stimulates the thymus gland, thereby helping the body to rid itself of infections and boosting the immune system.

This stone restores balance to the nerves, reducing stress and palpitations, and is also able to strengthen the heart and normalize its rhythm.

Orange Calcite

Orange calcite resonates with the sacral/abdomen chakra and is recommended for all problems of the reproductive system, particularly loss of libido.

An excellent stone for treating such digestive problems as constipation and irritable-bowel syndrome, it also cleanses the kidneys. Another of its benefits is its ability to release fear.

Red Calcite

Highly recommended for the base chakra, this energizing stone increases our vitality and zest for life.

Excellent for alleviating pain in the lower back, sciatica, and problems with the hips, legs, and knees, red calcite is also used to treat disorders of the reproductive organs on account of its ability to cleanse and stimulate the genitals. It may even be beneficial in cases of infertility.

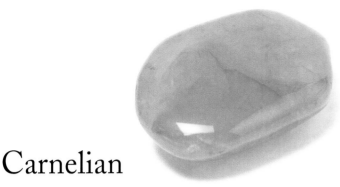

Carnelian

The most common colors of carnelian—a type of chalcedony that contains iron—are orange, orange-brown, red, and red-brown (also called "sard"), as well as the popular pink.

Tomb offerings carved from carnelian are prevalent in Egypt, revealing its importance as a protective stone for the ancient Egyptian dead. It is one of the stones that is believed to have been used in the breastplate of the Jewish high priest. During the Middle Ages carnelian was used to counteract rage.

HEALING PROPERTIES

Carnelian is particularly useful for the sacral, as well as the base, chakra, having the ability to boost fertility and stimulate sexuality and creativity. It is especially beneficial to those who find it difficult to express their sensuality.

Excellent for raising low energy levels and spurring the lethargic into action, carnelian stimulates the brain and clears the mind of confusion, thereby aiding concentration and problem-solving.

Carnelian is a stone of courage that makes us believe in, and stand up for, ourselves. By banishing negative emotions, such as fear and depression, carnelian protects and uplifts. Indeed, it may even be used to cleanse other stones.

Carnelian is recommended for treating disorders of the blood and circulation, particularly where there is a lack of warmth.

Charoite

An unmistakable stone that is found only in one location in Russia, charoite's colors include pink, lilac, lavender, violet, and purple.

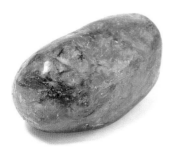

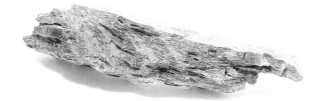

HEALING PROPERTIES

Charoite, which has a particular affinity for the brow, crown, and heart chakras, allows us to connect with the spiritual dimensions while still remaining grounded.

This stone is a magical and mysterious dream-fulfiller, with the ability to transform and manifest whatever it is that we want in our lives. A stone of prophecy, charoite assists us in understanding our visions.

Furthermore a cleanser and transmuter of negativity, charoite clears the aura and chakras by transforming any negativity into positive energy. It enables us to express our unconditional love by opening our hearts.

Because it encourages deep, peaceful sleep and allays nightmares, children may become very fond of this stone. Charoite also treats disorders of the eyes, heart, liver, and pancreas, as well as banishing headaches and alleviating aches and pains.

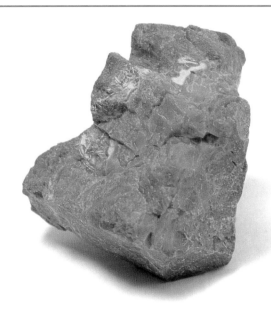

Chrysocolla

Chrysocolla is usually a bright blue-green color, although it can also be brown or black. Its name is derived from the Greek words *chrysos*, meaning "gold," and *kolla*, meaning "glue."

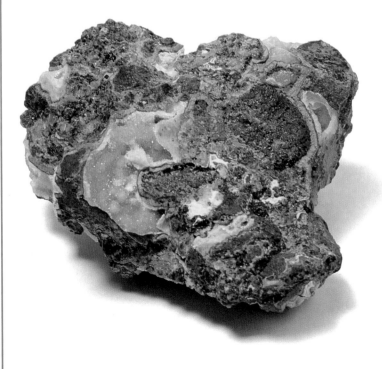

HEALING PROPERTIES

Chrysocolla has an affinity for the throat chakra and is therefore excellent for treating infections and inflammations of the sinuses, tonsils, larynx, and lungs. Because it assists communication and encourages us to speak our truth, chrysocolla promotes confidence and builds inner strength.

A cooling stone, chrysocolla soothes all types of inflammation, including burns, sunburn, and irritable-bowel syndrome, as well as helping one to keep a "cool" head.

Chrysocolla is a wonderful balancer, with the ability to regulate the nervous system, the heart, and the pancreas. It also works to balance the blood sugar and hormones (it can be used to relieve premenstrual tension and menstrual pain).

Further complaints that it helps to treat include all digestive upsets, such skeletal disorders as arthritis, muscular aches, pains, and spasms, ulcers, and blood disorders.

Finally, chrysocolla connects and aligns us with Mother Earth, encouraging us to appreciate the balance of nature and to seek to attain this balance within ourselves.

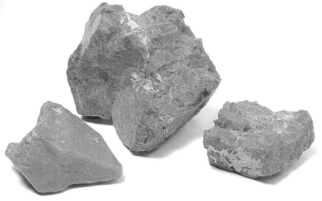

Chrysoprase

A vibrant, apple-green-colored type of chalcedony, chrysoprase was associated with the goddess Venus in Roman times.

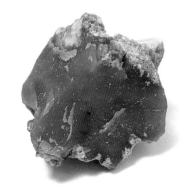

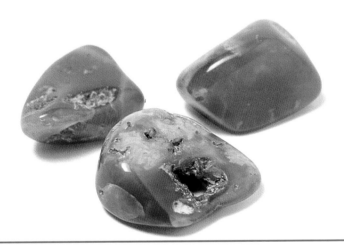

HEALING PROPERTIES

Chrysoprase has an affinity for the heart chakra, which it opens, activates, and energizes, giving it the ability to mend a broken heart, to heal relationships, and to transmute jealousy, envy, greed, selfishness, and grief into positive emotions.

A detoxifying stone, chrysoprase eliminates waste from the body, as well as the mind, by stimulating the liver and encouraging the body to rid itself of poisons. It furthermore promotes a peaceful night's sleep and is therefore ideal for children who suffer from nightmares.

Chrysoprase is also used to treat the reproductive organs, fertility problems, disorders of the lungs and thymus, and mental and physical exhaustion.

HEALING PROPERTIES

Citrine has a particular affinity for the solar-plexus chakra, which it cleanses and balances, encouraging wonder, delight, and enthusiasm. It is recommended for clearing the aura and filling any dark areas with happiness and light.

Marvelous for stimulating the brain and strengthening the intellect, citrine promotes new ideas and creativity and will enable you to solve problems more easily. Also known as a stone of abundance and prosperity, citrine can help you to acquire wealth, as well as to keep it.

An energizing stone that makes people feel good, citrine is ideal for those who are drained and tired and in need of an energy boost. It additionally benefits the kidneys, bladder, stomach, pancreas, and spleen.

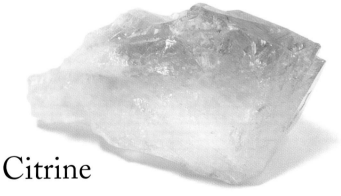

Citrine

Named after the French word *citron*, meaning "yellow," citrine is also known as yellow quartz. Its color varies from pale yellow to golden brown.

In ancient times, citrine was thought to protect against snake venom and evil thoughts. It was one of the stones that was incorporated into the breastplate of the Jewish high priest.

In common with azeztulite, citrine is unusual in that it never needs to be cleansed.

Danburite

Named for Danbury, Connecticut, where it was first found, danburite's color spectrum ranges from colorless through white to various shades of yellow and pink.

HEALING PROPERTIES

All types of danburite have an affinity for the crown chakra, while pink danburite is used to activate the heart chakra, opening the heart and encouraging us to trust once again.

Acting as a bridge between heaven and earth that links us with the divine consciousness, danburite is one of the most effective crystals for connecting with the angelic domain. Because it carries a very high vibration, it allows us to attain higher states of spirituality, thereby easing us along the pathway to enlightenment. Danburite is an excellent stone for releasing karma and helping us to make changes, thus enabling us to find our soul pathway.

Tremendous for balancing the right and left hemispheres of the brain and for releasing blockages in the acupuncture meridians, other uses of danburite include treating ailments of the liver and gallbladder and aiding the removal of toxins from the body, as well as the mind.

Diamond

The diamond's name is derived from the Greek word *adamas*, meaning "invincible," which refers to the fact that it is the hardest-known mineral and is impervious to scratching. As well as being colorless, diamonds can be white, black, yellow, red, pink, orange, brown, and green.

According to the Old Testament, diamonds appeared in the breastplate of the Jewish high priest. Throughout the ages the stone has variously been equated with Venus (the Roman goddess of love), justice, courage, and strength, and was once believed to be the ultimate protector.

Diamonds do not need to be recharged in crystal therapy.

HEALING PROPERTIES

Known as the "king of the crystals," the diamond has an affinity for the crown chakra. It is a stone of great purity that links us with the divine and removes any obstacles that lie before us on our pathway to enlightenment. Diamond is furthermore excellent for cleansing negativity from the aura.

Bestowing the qualities of perfection and innocence, diamond is a token of love. It helps to establish a strong and lasting relationship through its ability to urge couples to develop deep and everlasting trust and fidelity and to persevere and succeed in their relationships.

A stone that works to clear the mind, diamond enables one to see the necessary course of action clearly. It also treats dizziness and vertigo effectively.

Diamond may additionally be used to purify and detoxify all of the body's systems, to build up stamina, strength, and fearlessness, and to treat chronic conditions.

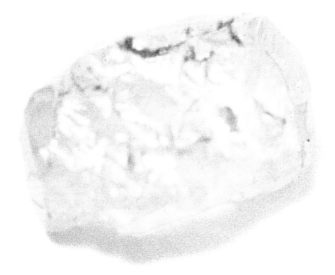

Emerald

Emerald is a form of beryl whose name is derived from the Greek word *beryllos*, which means "a green stone," and, indeed, its name describes its color: bright emerald green.

The Old Testament tells us that it was one of the stones that was used in the breastplate of the Jewish high priest.

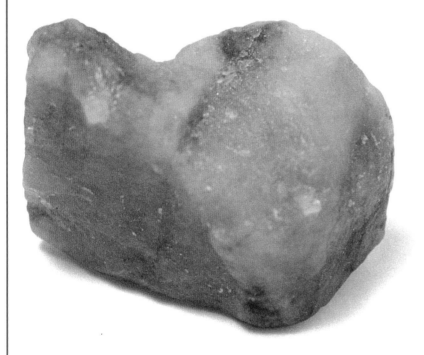

HEALING PROPERTIES

Emerald has an affinity for the heart chakra, which it opens and activates to heal all problems associated with the heart, whether they be physical or emotional. It is known as a stone of love with which unconditional love can be pledged to a partner.

By promoting harmony and wholeness in every aspect of one's life, emerald dispels negativity and draws beauty, wisdom, and healing to it. It encourages us to follow the laws of nature and, by imbuing us with a sense of beauty, openness, harmony, and balance, encourages us to appreciate the wonder of life.

Through its ability to stimulate the brain and enhance the memory, emerald guides us into making the right decisions. It is also an excellent stone for meditation because it facilitates deep breathing, relaxes the shoulders and upper back, and opens up the chest.

Emerald is highly beneficial in the treatment of all eye diseases. It is recommended that you place an emerald in a small bowl of water overnight and then soak absorbent-cotton pads in the emerald elixir and place them over your closed eyes.

Other therapeutic uses for emerald include alleviating spinal problems, muscular aches, skin ulcers, poor immune systems, liver complaints, and toxic conditions.

Fluorite

Fluorite (also known as fluorspar) is found in a variety of colors, including white, pink, magenta, purple, black, blue, green, and yellow. Its name is derived from the Latin verb *fluere*, which means "to be in a state of flux" or "to flow," reflecting its ease of melting and its use as a flux in metals. The word "fluorescent" is in turn derived from fluorite's name.

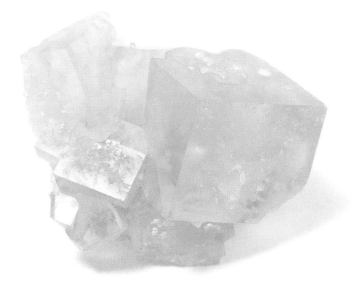

Yellow fluorite.

Purple fluorite.

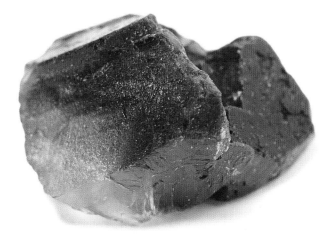

THE HEALING PROPERTIES OF SPECIFIC TYPES OF FLUORITE

The color of the stone will determine which chakra is balanced. Purple fluorite is excellent for activating the brow chakra. Green or pink fluorite aligns the heart chakra, and blue balances the throat chakra, while colorless fluorite stimulates the crown chakra.

Fluorite is an effective immune-booster that also stimulates the regeneration of cells, particularly in the skin and respiratory tract. Ulcers, cuts, and wounds, scars, herpes sores, and cankers will all benefit from treatment with fluorite. Indeed, fluorite is a stone that will discourage any disordered, chaotic growth.

Fluorite is generally used to improve the skeletal system's mobility. Blue fluorite is particularly beneficial for reducing inflammation as, for example, in rheumatoid arthritis. Fluorite furthermore has a harmonizing effect on the body on account of its ability to balance the nervous system, as well as bringing harmony and stability to relationships.

A stone that endows the mind with clarity and discernment, fluorite increases our powers of concentration and is therefore a useful study aid that enables us to absorb information rapidly. Purple fluorite is a wonderful stone for meditation that not only helps one to focus, but opens up the intuition and allows us to see through the veil of illusion. It enhances psychic ability, too.

Finally, fluorite is good for purification, whether it be of the body, the aura, or even a room.

Garnet

A crystal that derives its name from "pomegranate," there are many types of garnet, including almandine, andradite, grossularite, hessonite, melanite, pyrope, rhodolite, spessarite, and uvarovite. The color range is variable and includes shades of red, brown, black, orange, and green.

Garnet was used in the breastplate of the Jewish high priest. During the Middle Ages, warriors carried shields set with garnets to fill them with courage and protect them in battle.

HEALING PROPERTIES

Garnet has an affinity for the base chakra, where it breaks down blockages and stimulates the kundalini (our untapped creative energy). Garnet also keeps us grounded, making us feel safe and secure. It boosts our confidence and gives us the courage to face both everyday situations and crises. Garnet builds strength of character and enables us to find the inner strength needed to deal with life's challenges and to make necessary changes.

An excellent stone for stimulating the circulation and strengthening the heart, garnet is generally used to treat disorders of the blood. It additionally boosts the immune system, as well as energy levels, and is beneficial for those with spinal or joint problems.

Garnet is a stone of love and commitment that brings warmth, devotion, understanding, trust, sincerity, and honesty to a relationship. It can also help with any sexual difficulties.

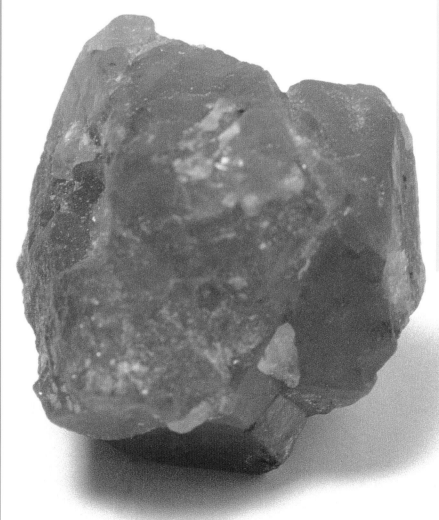

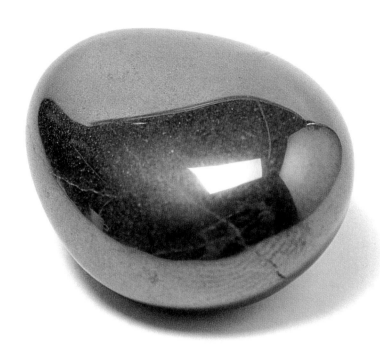

Hematite

Hematite is mainly black, gray, red, or reddish-brown in color. Its name is derived from the Greek word *haimatites*, which means "bloodlike" (an allusion to the vivid red color of the powdered stone). It was known as "bloodstone" during the Middle Ages.

Hematite was used for staunching the blood flow from wounds and for the formation of blood in Egypt.

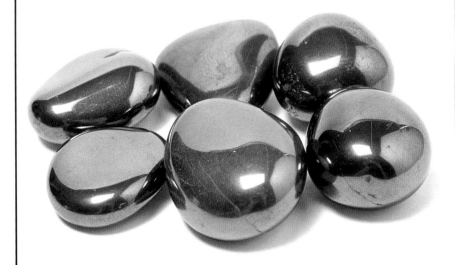

HEALING PROPERTIES

Hematite has an affinity for the base chakra and strengthens our connection with the earth, making us feel safe and secure and endowing us with courage, strength, endurance, and vitality. As well as helping to draw negativity from the base chakra and transmuting it, hematite will prevent you from absorbing the negativity of others, so carry a piece in your pocket to protect you.

A calming stone that helps to balance the nerves, you may use it to alleviate insomnia, stress, and anxiety. It is useful, too, at the end of a treatment for those who feel heady and ungrounded. Hematite also has the ability to keep you cool—mentally, as well as physically—so try placing it on the forehead to reduce a fever or on any painful or inflamed areas of the body to cool them.

Being traditionally associated with the blood, hematite is used to treat anemia in particular, although it will also improve the quality of the blood and reduce blood pressure. It is recommended for use during childbirth, partly to prevent excessive bleeding and partly to keep everyone calm. Sufferers of arthritis, leg cramps, and other musculoskeletal conditions may place a piece of hematite under their pillow to bring them relief.

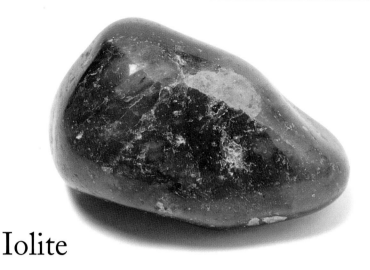

Iolite

Iolite (also known as cordierite) is a lovely blue to violet-blue stone that is often substituted for the more expensive blue sapphire, although it may also be blue, gray, green, or brown, its color appearing to change when viewed from different angles. Its name is derived from the Greek word *ios*, which means "violet."

HEALING PROPERTIES

Iolite has an affinity for the brow chakra. A wonderful stone for opening up the intuition, iolite is a stone of visions and dreams that has been used in shamanic healing ceremonies to enhance the gift of prophecy. It awakens our psychic abilities when used in meditation.

Iolite can be used to detoxify and rid the body of fatty deposits. Indeed, it may be beneficial to addictive personalities in general.

Jade

In the form of jadeite, jade's color ranges from white to green, but may also be pink, or, in the case of lavender jade, violet.

The ancients considered jade a sacred stone, and it was one of the crystals that was incorporated into the breastplate of the Jewish high priest. Jade was traditionally worn as a stone of good fortune, and was regarded as effective against kidney infections and stones.

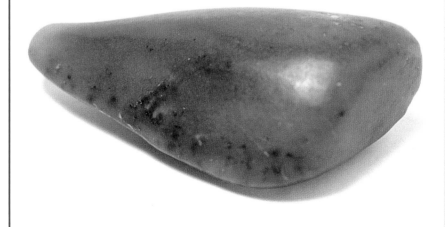

HEALING PROPERTIES

Both green and lavender jade have an affinity for the heart chakra, and both open up the heart on an emotional, as well as physical, level. Physically, jade is used for deepening the breathing and treating heart problems in general, whereas emotionally it encourages compassion and the establishment of strong bonds.

Jade balances the nervous system, dispelling mood swings and calming anger and irritability. Excellent for kidney problems, it also balances the metabolism.

It is also useful as a dream stone: a piece placed under the pillow will enable one both to remember and to interpret one's dreams. The stone of wisdom, jade helps us to reach decisions, too.

Jasper

Jasper is found in a variety of colors, of which brown, red, orange, yellow, and green are the most common.

Used for making amulets in Egypt, jasper was revered by ancient shamans as being a sacred and protective stone. It was one of the crystals that the Jewish high priest wore in his breastplate.

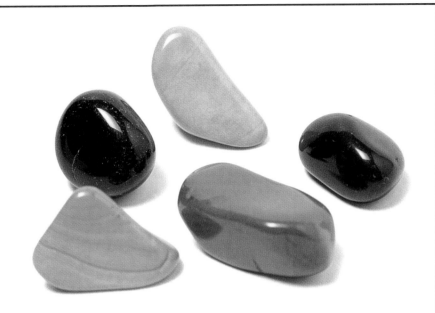

THE HEALING PROPERTIES OF SPECIFIC TYPES OF JASPER

Green Jasper (See Also Bloodstone)

Green jasper is a stone of balance that harmonizes the heart chakra. As well as helping to boost the immune system and detoxifying all of the body's systems, this stone protects against pollution.

Red Jasper

Red jasper balances and grounds the base chakra, bestowing courage and the willpower to achieve one's goals.

Excellent for stimulating the circulation and increasing energy, red jasper is a nurturing stone that is helpful in times of recovery. It may also be used to treat sexual problems and disorders of the intestines.

Yellow Jasper

Yellow jasper balances the solar-plexus chakra, calms the nerves, and is a useful protective stone. It also alleviates disorders of the stomach and relieves bloating.

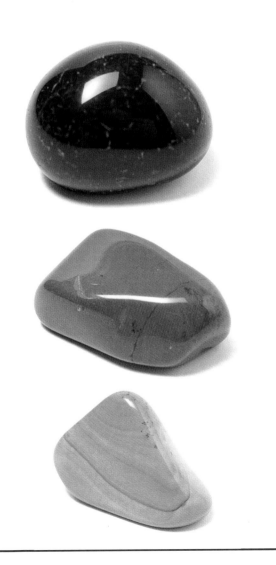

Kunzite

Kunzite is named after perhaps the world's greatest gem expert, Dr. George F. Kunz, who identified the stone. It is pale pink in hue, sometimes deepening to a pink-violet color.

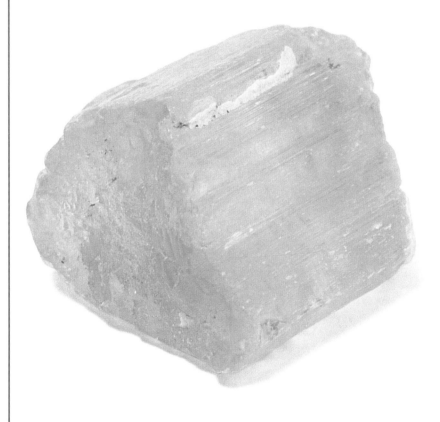

HEALING PROPERTIES

Kunzite has an affinity for the heart chakra, also aligning the heart with the throat and third-eye chakras. Exuding love, compassion, and peace, kunzite connects us with the unconditional love of the divine. This stone comforts and heals the heart on a physical, as well as an emotional, level, and is useful for those who find it difficult to express their emotions and bond with others. It also encourages the qualities of forgiveness and selfless devotion.

Kunzite is a protective stone that provides a shield against negative, unwanted energies. Having the power to raise our vibrations, it is a wonderful stone for meditation that allows one to reach a higher state of spiritual awareness and connect with the infinite source of love. It is excellent for enhancing the intuition, too.

Kunzite is ideal for babies and children, who are very attuned to the loving purity and innocence of this stone, which helps them to feel safe and secure.

Other uses for kunzite include dissolving panic attacks and relieving stress and tension, as well as treating lung disease, circulatory problems, sciatica, neuralgia, and hormonal problems.

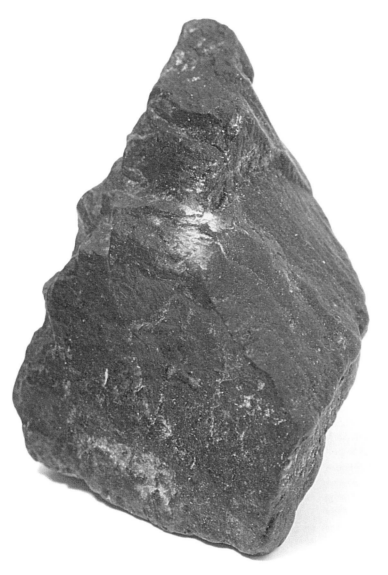

Lapis lazuli

It is thought that lapis lazuli's name is derived from the Latin word *lapis*, meaning "stone," and the Persian *lazur*, meaning "blue."

Highly prized by the ancients, the Egyptians used it in their temples because they believed that it was a stone from heaven (its midnight-blue color recalls the sky and its flecks of pyrite resemble the stars). One of the stones that featured in the breastplate of the Jewish high priest, the Hebrews decorated their robes of ceremony with lapis lazuli, while the tablets on which Moses received the law were reputedly made of this stone. It is said to have been given to humankind by the angels.

HEALING PROPERTIES

Lapis lazuli has a particular affinity for both the third-eye and throat chakras. When placed on the third-eye chakra, it connects us with the source of omnipotence and reveals our inner truth. Lapis lazuli heightens and expands our attunement to the intuitive, encouraging psychic development and introducing visions and insights into our dreams. If placed on the throat chakra, lapis lazuli opens up and energizes this center. Extensively used to treat disorders of the throat, thyroid, neck, vocal cords, ears, chest, and lungs, it cools and soothes areas of inflammation and boosts the immune system to encourage a speedy recovery.

Lapis lazuli is excellent for dispelling repressed anger and balancing mood swings. It is recommended that those who find it difficult to speak out and express their emotions use it because it encourages one to speak one's truth and inspires confidence. This stone brings mental clarity, too, as well as providing clarity in verbal communication.

Lapis lazuli is a stone of protection that may be worn to guard against psychic attacks. Other uses for it include reducing pain, inducing a good night's sleep, relieving vertigo and dizziness, and promoting purification.

Larimar

Also known as blue pectolite, the dolphin stone, or the Atlantis stone, larimar is usually a pale-blue to medium-blue color, although it can also be white, red, or green. Larimar was discovered in the Bahamas and the Dominican Republic about twenty years ago.

HEALING PROPERTIES

Along with the throat chakra, larimar has an affinity for the third-eye and heart chakras. As well as helping to heal and tone the throat, larimar opens up the throat chakra, thereby promoting self-confidence and encouraging us to express our deepest fears and truths.

Larimar is used as a meditation stone because it quickly calms the mind and bestows inner peace, also facilitating contact with the angelic realms and bringing forth past lives from Atlantis. It therefore blesses us with insights into the secrets of the universe.

A stone of harmony, larimar assists in balancing the yin-yang energies and thus in unifying our male and female qualities. It is excellent for unplugging the meridians and dissolving energy blocks, particularly in the head, neck, and chest.

Larimar embraces love and joy, opening up the heart by allowing us to express unconditional love and to play like children.

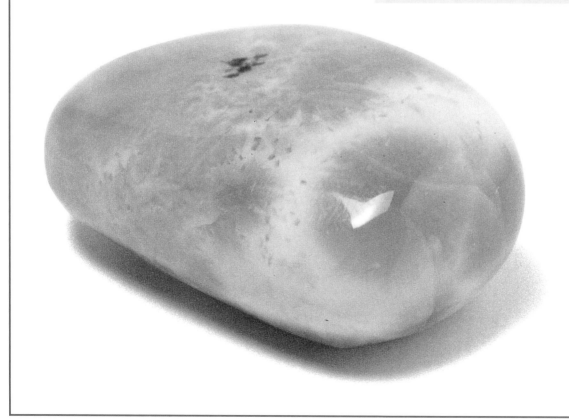

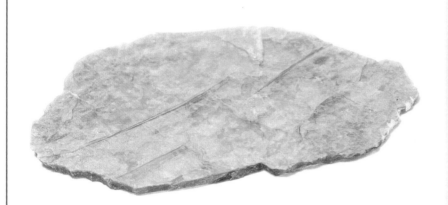

Lepidolite

Lepidolite, which ranges from pink to violet in color, has only become available in large quantities on the mineral market during the past decade. Its name, derived from the Greek, means "scale stone."

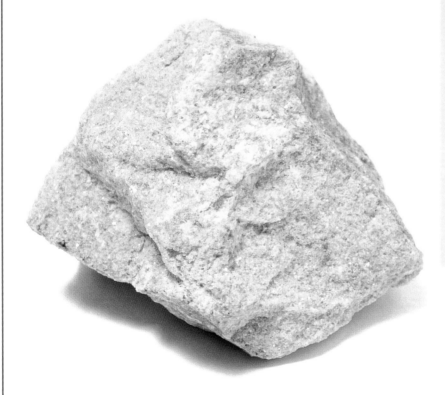

HEALING PROPERTIES

Although lepidolite has a particular affinity for the third-eye and crown chakras, it is also useful for activating the heart and throat chakras.

An excellent stone for meditation, as well as for treating sleep disturbances, lepidolite calms the mind and is most beneficial for relieving stress and tension. It also relieves tightness in the muscles and alleviates nerve pain, such as sciatica and neuralgia.

Because it helps us to concentrate and focus on the tasks before us, lepidolite encourages decision-making and clarity of thought. It may be used to treat people in confused states of mind: those suffering from Alzheimer's disease, for example, or recovering from an anesthetic.

Lepidolite helps both to induce change and to support us through periods of change. Allowing us to release our old patterns and move on, lepidolite even eases the transition from this life to the next world.

Lepidolite can be used for earth healing on account of the stability that it provides for the ley lines and tectonic plates. It furthermore promotes a calm environment and protects us against electromagnetic influences.

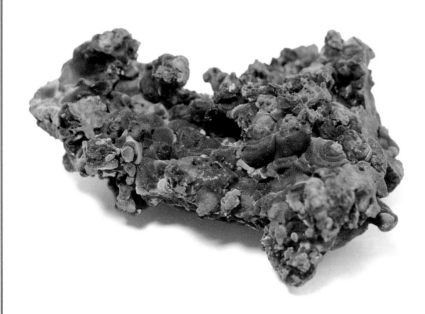

Malachite

Malachite ranges from light to dark green in color.

A stone steeped in history, it was extensively used in Egypt, where it was dedicated to the goddess Hathor. It was also sacred to the Roman goddess Venus and the Norse goddess Freya. During the Middle Ages it was a popular remedy for menstrual problems and labor pain and is therefore sometimes called the "midwife stone."

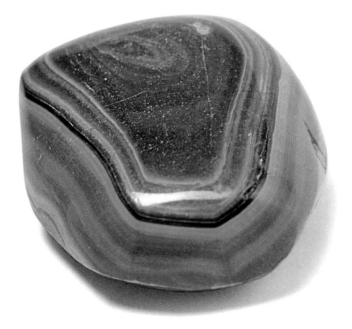

HEALING PROPERTIES

Malachite, which has an affinity for the heart and throat chakras, is a stone of balance that soothes, yet also strengthens, the nervous system. Malachite will balance mood swings and attune you to the beauty and healing greenness of nature. Excellent for the heart, it draws out past hurts and heals them and will similarly replace depression with peace and tranquillity. It has the power to bring fidelity to a relationship and loyalty to a friendship.

A stone of change and transformation, malachite encourages old traumas and negative experiences from the past to come to the surface, where they can be released to enable us to move on and realize our goals.

Malachite has excellent healing powers. Not only does it boost the immune system, making us less susceptible to illness, but if a disease has already taken hold, it stimulates regeneration and rejuvenation, thereby speeding up recovery. Beneficial for the muscles and joints, malachite bestows flexibility on the limbs, relieves cramps, reduces swellings, and promotes the healing of bones. As evidenced by its alternative name, the "midwife stone," it facilitates labor, also alleviating such menstrual disorders as P.M.T. and period pains, as well as the menopause.

Finally, malachite is a detoxifying stone that cleanses the body of physical and emotional impurities.

Morganite

Morganite is a rose-pink-colored variety of beryl, the "mother of gemstones." It was discovered this century by John Morgan, the noted American industrialist after whom the stone is named.

HEALING PROPERTIES

Morganite—a symbol of unconditional love—has a strong affinity for the heart chakra, which it cleanses and activates. Because it attracts love to those who wear it, and maintains love within a relationship, it is excellent for those who feel rejected and unloved. Deep healing can occur if morganite is placed on the heart chakra, enabling one to let go of hurtful past experiences.

Morganite is a profoundly relaxing stone that gently soothes away all states of anxiety. It is recommended that those who suffer from such symptoms as palpitations, hyperventilation, and panic attacks carry a piece of morganite to stabilize and calm their heart and lungs. Sexual problems, such as impotence and frigidity, may also respond to morganite's healing touch.

Highly beneficial as a meditative aid, holding a piece of morganite or sitting in a morganite circle will draw to us the ascended master Lady Kwan Yin, the mother of compassion. Kwan Yin fills us with universal love, healing, and patience, guiding us toward a more contemplative lifestyle and making us aware of the pointlessness of materialism and of the importance of our spirituality. Morganite encourages a simple, childlike view of the world.

Obsidian

Obsidian, which is formed by the rapid cooling of volcanic lava, is also called "rock glass" or "volcanic glass" because it is created so rapidly that there is no time for facets to be formed. Obsidian derives its name from its discoverer, Obsius, who, according to the prominent Roman historian, Pliny the Elder, found the stone in present-day Ethiopia. The color is usually black, silvery, or brown, but may also be blue, green, purple, or red.

Obsidian is easily broken into sharp-edged pieces, and these obsidian flakes were used by ancient humankind as spearheads and tools. Obsidian was prized by the Aztecs, and the Mayan priests of the god Tezcatlipoca ("Smoking Mirror") employed obsidian for scrying to predict the future. It was believed in antiquity that obsidian could drive out demons.

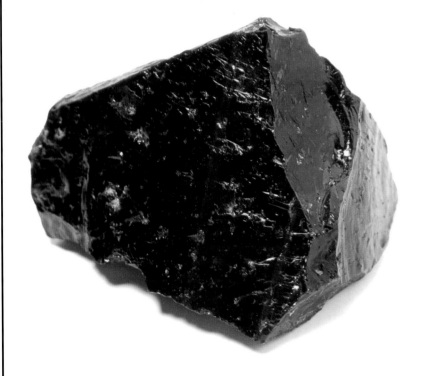

HEALING PROPERTIES

Obsidian has an affinity for the base chakra and is an excellent stone for grounding and anchoring us firmly to Mother Earth, making us feel stable and balanced.

Obsidian represents eternal protection and will shield the wearer from physical, emotional, or psychic attack. It will purify a negative atmosphere and purge negativity from dysfunctional chakras and meridians. Obsidian can also remove toxins from the body, as well as from polluted areas of the Earth.

Polished balls of obsidian may be used for scrying, the glassy surface not only reflecting our future, but the dark, "shadow" parts of ourselves, thereby enabling us to discover our true nature. The truth can hurt, however, and obsidian confronts us with our deepest fears, pain, and energy blocks. Although we may find this uncomfortable, obsidian releases us from the shadow's grip, bringing peace and light where there was once darkness.

An excellent stone for pain relief, obsidian is used to treat joint pain, such as that caused by arthritis, and to alleviate muscular aches and spasms. It also improves circulation and is tremendous for those suffering from hardening of the arteries. Obsidian can furthermore remove the shock and trauma that arise after an injury has been sustained.

Peridot

Peridot (pronounced "pair-a-doe"), which is also known as olivine or chrysolite, is formed from the magma in volcanic rock. It is usually bottle, olive, or yellowish-green in color.

Peridot was worn as jewelry by the ancient Egyptians, who also employed it for healing purposes. It has been mined as a gemstone for an estimated four thousand years and is mentioned in the Bible, where it is called by the Hebrew name *pitdah*, also being said to have been one of the stones that was used in the breastplate of the Jewish high priest. Peridot was used to drive away evil spirits during the Middle Ages.

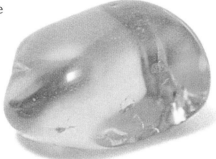

HEALING PROPERTIES

Peridot, which has an affinity for the heart chakra, has the power to cleanse the heart of jealousy, resentment, bitterness, hatred, and greed, enabling us to forgive and forget and opening up our hearts to joy and new relationships. A stone for releasing anger and guilt, it is excellent for detoxifying the liver, which may store these emotions, as well as the gallbladder.

Peridot provides a shield of protection that prevents others from draining our precious energy. A generally revitalizing and energizing stone, it may be employed to banish lethargy, apathy, and exhaustion. Indeed, peridot works as a good overall tonic for the body, strengthening the immune system and preventing illnesses from recurring. It may be used for disorders of the lungs, too, on account of its ability to encourage the body to disperse mucus. Peridot may also strengthen the eyesight and heal digestive complaints and skin problems, particularly warts.

Phenacite

Phenacite's name is derived from the Greek word *phenakos*, which means "deceiver" (referring to the fact that it is often mistaken for quartz). Its color spectrum ranges from colorless through white and yellow, to pink, pale red, and brown.

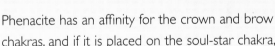

HEALING PROPERTIES

Phenacite has an affinity for the crown and brow chakras, and if it is placed on the soul-star chakra, above the crown chakra, an immediate activation can be detected. A stone of the higher dimensions, with a very elevated vibration, it is a powerful stone for meditation. Phenacite enables us to focus on our spiritual side and accelerates our spiritual ascension by expanding our consciousness and allowing us to access, and communicate with, our angels and guides.

Phenacite has the ability to heal all levels of our being. When used with other stones in crystal therapy, phenacite greatly enhances the effectiveness of their healing powers.

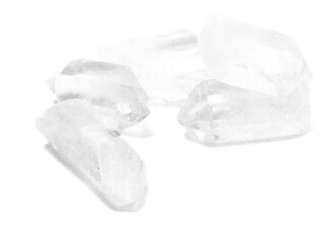

Clear Quartz

It is said that quartz crystals were used in Atlantis and Lemuria for rejuvenation, while ancient priests used it to destroy negative energy. The ancient Greeks believed that it was water that had been frozen by their gods and therefore called it *Krystallos*, meaning "ice." As well as carrying them in the summer to keep their hands cool, the Romans used quartz crystals to give pain relief and to treat fevers and swellings. Similarly, during the Middle Ages, a quartz crystal was placed on the tongue to reduce a fever. Clear quartz is extensively used for healing today.

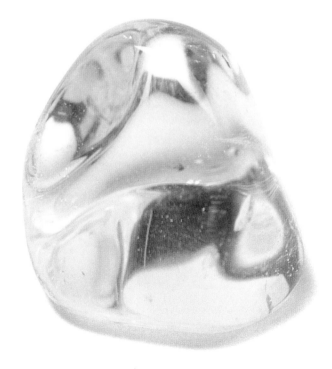

HEALING PROPERTIES

Known as the "master healer," clear quartz may be programed for any purpose and will amplify the effect of other crystals. Kirlian photography has revealed that when a quartz crystal is held in the hand, the strength of the energy field is at least doubled. It therefore follows that placing one on any part of the body will increase the energy in that area.

Clear quartz can furthermore be used to stabilize any chakra and may be used on the crown chakra to bring clarity to meditation and dreams. (The crystal balls that are used for scrying are usually made of clear quartz.)

In summary, quartz clears blockages and balances and revitalizes the physical, mental, emotional, and spiritual planes, as well as bestowing clarity and increasing energy fields. It is recommended that you always carry or wear a piece of clear quartz, which will both protect you and enable you to maintain your balance. A piece of clear crystal is also a must for the home and work environments.

Specific Types of Quartz

Aqua Aura Quartz

These are clear quartz crystals that have been combined with pure gold.

HEALING PROPERTIES

Aqua aura quartz is used to stimulate the throat chakra in particular, but will also activate all of the chakras, cleanse the aura, and eliminate negativity. It has the power to boost the immune system, too.

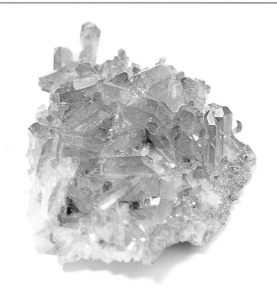

Green Quartz

This quartz crystal is green in color.

HEALING PROPERTIES

Green quartz opens, activates, and balances the heart chakra. It dissolves past hurts, resentments, envy, and bitterness, replacing such negative emotions with everlasting, unconditional love.

Rose Quartz

Rose quartz, which is found in various shades of pink, has been used for centuries to heal the heart and to treat fertility problems.

HEALING PROPERTIES

With its affinity for the heart chakra, rose quartz has the power to fill us with a sense of unconditional love, for ourselves, as well as for others. By enabling us to give and receive love, rose quartz encourages us to overcome emotional traumas and to develop a spirit of forgiveness and trust.

A stone of gentleness and calm, rose quartz balances all of the body's systems, reducing high blood pressure, strengthening and balancing the heart, and restoring a sense of peace and tranquillity. It is an excellent stone for bringing harmony to a chaotic situation.

Finally, rose quartz has the power to increase fertility: I have seen it work many times!

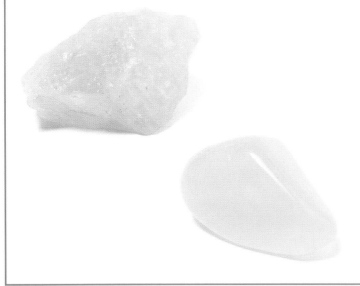

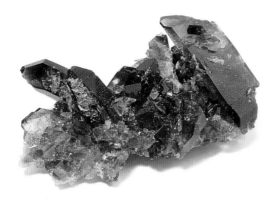

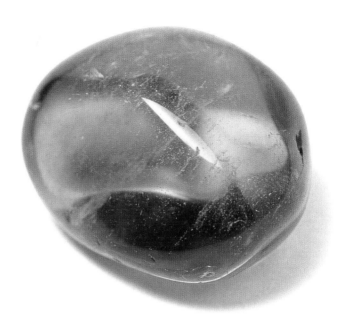

Smoky Quartz

Smoky quartz is either a smoky light to dark brown, gray, or black in color.

In the past, it was often worn or carried by solders for protection.

HEALING PROPERTIES

Smoky quartz has an affinity for the solar-plexus chakra and is an excellent grounding stone that is often used at the end of a treatment.

Beneficial for relieving stress and anxiety, smoky quartz calms a hyperactive mind, disperses fear, lifts depression and negativity, and encourages positive thoughts and action.

As well as being a detoxifying stone that prompts elimination, especially of the digestive system, smoky quartz protects us against radiation and other dangers. It is a pain-relieving stone that alleviates back pain and eases muscular spasms.

Tangerine Quartz

This quartz is tangerine in color.

HEALING PROPERTIES

Tangerine quartz has an affinity for the sacral chakra, making it useful for treating any sexual problem, including impotence, frigidity, and infertility.

Tangerine quartz is also an excellent stone to employ following a shock or trauma. If an injury has been sustained, it will restore the energy flow to the affected area. This stone will additionally alleviate kidney, bladder, and intestinal disorders.

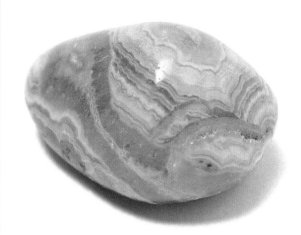

Rhodochrosite

Also known as raspberry or manganese spar, rhodochrosite (whose name is derived from the Greek for "rose colored") is a striking raspberry-pink color.

HEALING PROPERTIES

Rhodochrosite has an affinity for the heart chakra. On a physical level, it regulates the heart beat, stabilizing the pulse rate, balances the blood pressure, and stimulates the circulation. On an emotional level, rhodochrosite opens up the heart, lifting depression and encouraging a positive, cheerful attitude to life. Because it prompts spontaneity, it is ideal for those who find it difficult to express their feelings. A stone of love and passion, rhodochrosite is believed to have the power to attract one's soul mate.

Rhodochrosite additionally stimulates the mind and encourages creativity and innovation. Its other properties include the ability to alleviate migraines, skin disorders, and thyroid imbalances, as well as kidney and intestinal problems.

Rhodonite

Rhodonite is named after the Greek *rhodos,* meaning "rose colored." It is rose-pink, usually with black veins of manganese dioxide, but may also be yellow, brownish-red, or black.

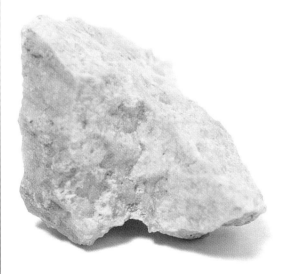

HEALING PROPERTIES

Rhodonite has a strong affinity for the heart chakra. It encourages us to forgive and forget our past traumas, allowing the heart chakra to heal. Rhodonite is a stone of compassion that enables us to express the purity of unconditional love toward ourselves, as well as others.

Rhodonite helps to dispel anxiety, fears, and panic attacks. It may be used as soon as possible after traumatic events to bring balance, calmness, and harmony to the recipient. Where such feelings as bitterness, jealousy, anger, selfishness, and depression have been suppressed, rhodonite allows them to rise to the surface to be released.

Rhodonite is excellent for cuts, wounds, and insect bites. It draws such toxins as pus to the surface for rapid healing. This stone boosts fertility and stimulates the libido. Heart disorders will also benefit.

Ruby

Reflecting its color range of pinkish-red to red, the ruby's name is derived from the Latin word *rubeus*, which means "red."

The ancients considered the ruby to be the stone of the sun and believed that it represented the life force and fire. It was one of the stones that was incorporated into the breastplate of the Jewish high priest.

HEALING PROPERTIES

Ruby has an affinity for the base chakra, which its strong energy sparks into life, spurring lethargy into action and eliminating apathy and exhaustion. Because it also increases sexual activity, its use is indicated for the treatment of impotence and frigidity. Ruby stimulates the heart chakra, too, filling our hearts with joy, spontaneity, laughter, and courage. It instills in us a great passion and zest for life, as well as confidence.

Finally, as its blood-red color suggests, it is excellent for improving the circulation and quality of the blood.

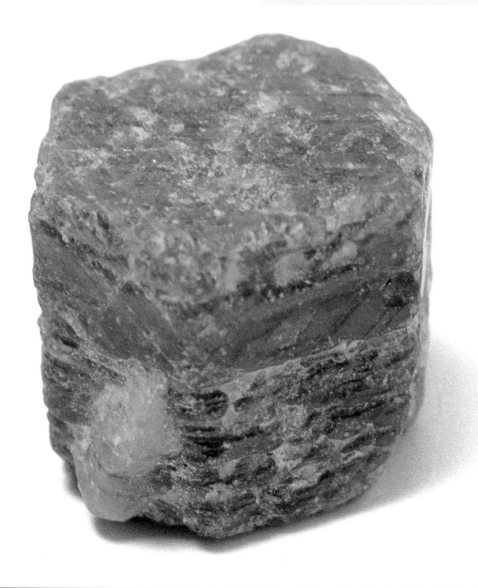

Sapphire

Sapphire is found in a variety of colors, including blue, yellow, white, black, purple, and green. Its name is derived from the Sanskrit word *Sani*, which means "Saturn."

Sapphire has always been associated with love, joy, prosperity, fidelity, the heavens, and the angels. It is said to have been one of the stones in the breastplate of the Jewish high priest.

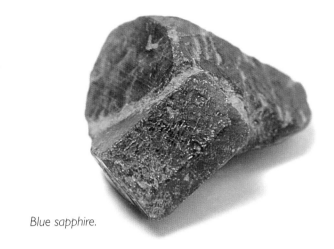

Blue sapphire.

The Healing Properties of Specific Types of Sapphire

Black Sapphire

Black sapphire is a stone for protection and grounding.

Blue Sapphire

Because blue sapphire has a particular affinity for the throat chakra, it prompts you to express your truth and beliefs. As well as encouraging communication and helping those engaged in public speaking, it has physical benefits for the throat, thyroid, parathyroid, and lungs.

Blue sapphire has a calming and balancing effect on the nervous system. It may also be used as a meditation aid to open up the crown and brow chakras to the angelic realms. Some sapphires are believed to be record-keepers and may aid you to access the knowledge of ancient civilizations when dreaming or meditating.

Green Sapphire

Green sapphire helps to balance the heart chakra and boosts the immune system.

Indigo Sapphire

Indigo sapphire activates the third-eye chakra, enhancing psychic awareness.

Pink Sapphire

Pink sapphire fills the heart chakra with unconditional love and peace.

Purple Sapphire

Purple sapphire awakens the crown chakra, encouraging you along the path to enlightenment.

Yellow Sapphire

Yellow sapphire balances and activates the solar-plexus chakra, clearing the mind of negativity, stimulating the intellect, and bringing wisdom.

A detoxifying stone, yellow sapphire rids the body of impurities and stimulates the lymphatic system. Liver and gallbladder problems in particular will benefit from its use.

Yellow sapphire is furthermore associated with wealth and prosperity and is identified with the Hindu god Ganesh, who is a remover of obstacles. It is worn by some merchants in the Far East to attract wealth and obtain the fulfillment of their ambitions.

White Sapphire

White sapphire enhances the crown chakra, establishing a close connection with the heavens and angelic spheres.

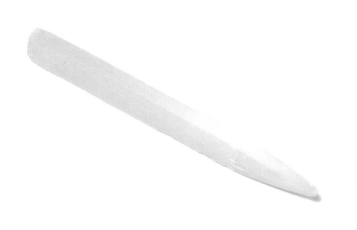

Selenite

Selenite is usually white or colorless, but may also be pink or sandy in color. It is said to be under the influence of Selene, the Roman goddess of the full moon, for whom it is named.

HEALING PROPERTIES

Selenite has an affinity for the crown chakra, making it an excellent tool for meditation that allows you to access both past and future lives. Simply rub your stone while in a meditative state and take note of any visual images or symbols that may appear, or feelings that you may experience.

Because selenite has a very high vibration, it is a wonderful stone for healing, of both physical and emotional ailments. Promoting flexibility of the mind, as well as of the body (it strengthens the spine and increases its suppleness), it encourages us to broaden our horizons and to go with the flow.

As well as acting against other toxins, selenite helps to prevent the damage caused by mercury fillings in the teeth. It has the power to stimulate cellular regeneration and may even increase one's life span.

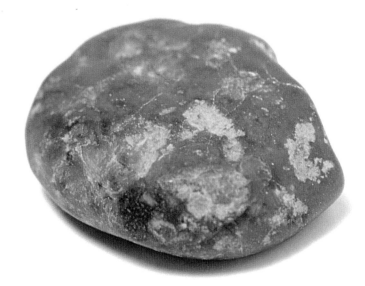

Shattuckite

An unusual stone that is light to dark blue. It is named after the location where it was found: the Shattuck mine in Arizona.

HEALING PROPERTIES

Shattuckite has an affinity for the throat and the third-eye chakras. It clears the throat area, alleviating such physical conditions as tonsillitis and laryngitis, and encourages us to speak our truth. Shattuckite is an excellent stone for channeling, enabling us to verbalize clearly the information being received from the other worlds. It also provides protection during channeling.

Shattuckite stimulates the third eye to open up our intuition and to clarify any psychic visions.

Sugilite

Sugilite is named after Dr. Ken-ichi Sugi, the Japanese geologist who discovered the first specimens of the stone in 1944. Also known as iuvilite, royal azel, and new-age stone, sugilite's color spectrum ranges from deep lavender to purple.

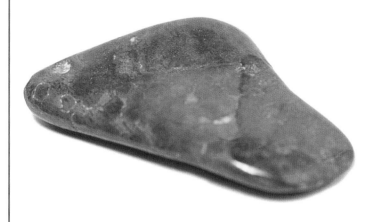

HEALING PROPERTIES

Sugilite has an affinity for the brow, crown, and heart chakras. With its power to enhance the intuition and to encourage the development of psychic ability, this stone both makes us believe in our sixth sense and strengthens it. Because it connects us with the pure love of the divine, sugilite is a wonderful stone to use for meditation.

Another of sugilite's uses is to protect sensitive souls. Helpful for grounding, and with the ability to enable us to understand the reasons why we are on the Earthly plane and the lessons that we are here to learn, it is ideal for those who feel that they do not belong in this world. A nurturing stone that helps us to confront unpleasant situations and fears, it encourages us to accept what we must face.

Sugilite is an excellent pain-reliever that will draw out pain when placed on affected areas.

HEALING PROPERTIES

Yellow sunstone has an affinity for the solar-plexus chakra and removes stress, anxiety, and fear from this energy center, suffusing it with light. An uplifting crystal, yellow sunstone fills you with love and laughter, as well as increasing your confidence, boosting your self-esteem, and inspiring optimism. In crystal therapy, yellow sunstone is furthermore used to treat eating disorders and to encourage weight loss.

Because orange sunstone has an affinity for the sacral chakra, it is excellent for treating sexual problems and disorders of the reproductive organs. This stone also cleanses the kidneys, bladder, and intestines, and alleviates spinal problems.

Sunstone

The two main types of sunstone are orange sunstone and a yellow sunstone (sometimes known as golden labradorite) that comes from the American state of Oregon.

This stone represented the sun god in ancient Greece, while in India it was believed to provide protection. It is placed in the center of the wheel in Native American rituals of the medicine wheel, when it is said to glow.

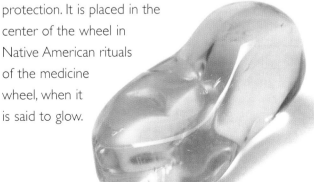

Tanzanite

An uncommon mineral, tanzanite was discovered in Tanzania (after which it is named) in 1967. Since then, it has been widely used in crystal therapy. A variety of zoisite, tanzanite's color ranges from clear through yellowish-brown, green, and blue to purple. The blue-lavender tanzanite is particularly therapeutic.

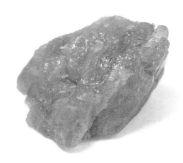

HEALING PROPERTIES

Tanzanite has an affinity for the brow and crown chakras, as well as for the throat chakra. By activating our psychic abilities and raising our vibratory rate, it facilitates communication with the spiritual world, enabling us to link with angelic beings, ascended masters, guides, and other spiritual beings from other dimensions. In addition, tanzanite allows us to receive visions from the spiritual world.

A stone of transformation that dissolves old patterns of disease and karma, tanzanite enables us to move forward with optimism and inspiration, giving us a sense of direction and allowing us to manifest our powers for the highest good.

Tanzanite enhances healing at all levels, as well as protecting those who are doing the healing. It works particularly well with iolite, kunzite, phenacite, and morganite when raising vibrations. Physically, tanzanite clears the throat and lungs and alleviates disorders of the skin, ears, and eyes. It boosts the immune system, speeding up recovery after an illness, and detoxifies and regenerates cells and tissues. Further uses for tanzanite include treating spinal problems and diseases of the reproductive system.

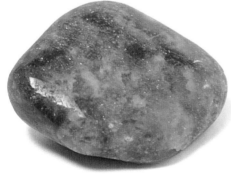

Thulite

A variety of zoisite, thulite's name is derived from the legendary island of Thule that is described in Germanic lore. Pinkish-red-colored thulite is particularly therapeutic, but it may also be green, yellow, or gray.

HEALING PROPERTIES

Thulite is particularly suitable for use with the heart, third-eye, and sacral chakras. By helping to activate the heart chakra, it enables us to express unconditional love and allows us both to give and receive love, making it excellent for those who have experienced hurtful relationships.

Thulite is a helpful stone for those who are weak because it bestows strength and energy upon the wearer. It also gives us a sense of adventure.

Physically, thulite may be used to treat heart disease and breathing problems (especially asthma) and accelerates recovery times. A beneficial stone for the reproductive organs, thulite may also be used to alleviate sexual problems and to enhance the libido, as well as fertility.

Tiger's Eye

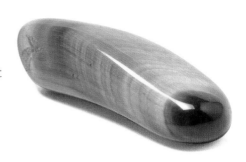

Tiger's eye is a variety of quartz. It is formed when quartz crystals replace crocidolite fibers (mineral-bearing asbestos), which reflect the light and exhibit a chatoyancy (cat's-eye) effect. Tiger's eye is most commonly golden-brown in color, but may also be red, blue, or black.

Traditionally used to attract wealth, abundance, and good luck, during the Middle Ages this stone was worn to ward off the evil eye and witchcraft.

HEALING PROPERTIES

Tiger's eye has a particular affinity for the solar-plexus chakra. Its gold and brown colors bring together the energies of heaven and Earth, enabling us to lift our vibrations while at the same time feeling grounded and stable.

Recommended as a protective stone, tiger's eye dispels fear and anxiety and counteracts feelings of hypochondria, making it an excellent antidote to psychosomatic illnesses. With its ability to imbue us with will-power, purpose, courage, and self-confidence, it additionally balances mood swings, as well as our yin-yang energies, and releases tension.

Tiger's eye furthermore encourages mental clarity, allowing us to see a problem objectively, unclouded by emotions. It may therefore be used when our ideas are confused, helping us to see our goals clearly and to make the right decisions.

Other uses for tiger's eye include treating neck and throat disorders, eye problems, and reproductive diseases, as well as strengthening the spinal column, releasing toxins, and alleviating pain.

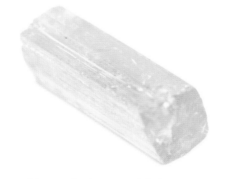

Topaz

Topaz can be yellow, brown, blue, colorless, or pink. It was one of the stones used in the breastplate of the Jewish high priest. The ancient Egyptians connected the stone with the sun god, Ra. In India and Europe, topaz was associated with the planet Jupiter. In Mexico, topaz was used to ascertain the truth. African Bushmen use it in their ceremonies to communicate with the spirit world and to attract and manifest both wealth and health.

HEALING PROPERTIES

Topaz has an affinity for the abdomen and solar-plexus chakras. It is a wonderful aid for increasing vitality. Topaz stimulates and unblocks the meridians and speeds up a sluggish metabolism. Feelings of uncertainly are dispelled and confidence and trust in oneself are magnified.

Topaz is an excellent stone for attraction and manifestation. It attracts people to you on both friendship and business levels. Topaz enables you to manifest your desires, as long as they are for the greater good.

Topaz can be used for such eating disorders as loss of appetite, anorexia, bulimia, and obesity since it balances the solar-plexus and abdomen chakras. It may also help to heal skin problems.

Tourmaline

There are many varieties of tourmaline, including achroite (colorless), buergerite (dark brown to black), dravite (brown), elbaite (all colors, including red, pink, green, blue, orange, and yellow), indicolite (blue), rubellite (red, violet, and pink), verdelite (green), schorl (black), and uvite (light to dark brown). It is therefore apt that tourmaline's name is derived from the Singhalese word *tourmali*, meaning "mixed colored stones."

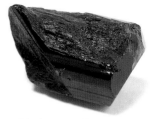

Black tourmaline.

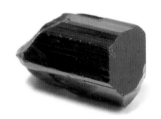

HEALING PROPERTIES

Tourmaline offers many healing benefits for all of the body's systems, while its various colors may be used to balance all of the chakras.

Black Tourmaline

Black tourmaline is excellent when used as a grounding stone after a treatment and also balances those who feel "spaced out."

A powerful protector against the negative energy that emanates from other individuals, be it from the Earthly or spirit plane, if used with mica, black tourmaline will reflect negative energy, returning it to the sender. It also deflects negative energy from electrical equipment and neutralizes the effects of radiation.

An energy-enhancer that increases feelings of vitality and well-being and lifts the spirits, this stone may be used to treat lower-back problems and adrenal disorders, also providing pain relief.

Blue Tourmaline

Blue tourmaline activates the throat and third-eye chakras, making it excellent for treating disorders of the throat, lungs, and eyes.

As well as increasing communication and opening up the intuition to enable contact with the spiritual realms, blue tourmaline facilitates the release of suppressed grief.

This stone also has the power to cool and heal burns.

Green Tourmaline

Green tourmaline has an affinity for the heart chakra, which it opens and fills with love and compassion. A stone of release that encourages emotional issues to rise to the surface so that they can be released, it can also rid you of past-life traumas and physical toxins.

Green tourmaline balances the emotions, thereby dissolving stress and fear and inducing sleep and tranquillity. It can be used to treat problems of the heart, thymus, and immune system, as well as to aid weight loss.

Pink Tourmaline

An excellent stone for the heart chakra, which it suffuses with love and joy, pink tourmaline is often given as a token of friendship or love.

A deeply relaxing stone that makes us feel peaceful and secure, pink tourmaline is a good choice for anyone who has been physically abused. It also has the power to comfort those who have been recently bereaved.

On a physical level, pink tourmaline may be used to treat the heart, lungs, and skin.

Yellow Tourmaline

This stone activates the solar-plexus chakra, stimulating creativity and the intellect, bestowing clarity of mind, and increasing feelings of courage and personal power. All in all, yellow tourmaline is an excellent crystal for those in business.

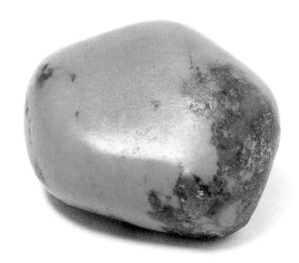

Turquoise

Turquoise is, of course, turquoise in color, although its hue may vary from greenish- to sky-blue. Black, brown, or gold veins usually run through the stone.

A very ancient and powerful stone, turquoise was mined from at least 6000 B.C. by the early Egyptians. Greatly revered as a sacred stone by Tibetan shamans, as well as in India and the Middle East, North American shamans used it to initiate rain. Many cultures consider it to be a protective stone that bestows health and strength upon the wearer.

HEALING PROPERTIES

Although turquoise has a particular affinity for the throat, heart, and brow chakras, it may be employed to align and balance all of the chakras and meridians. An excellent cleansing stone for the throat chakra, turquoise can help to soothe and clear sore throats, as well as to purify the lungs. It encourages both oral and written communication and the expression of one's true feelings.

A stone of balance, turquoise is tremendous for stabilizing mood swings and calming the nerves. It has the power to prevent panic attacks and aids recovery following a nervous breakdown.

Turquoise may be worn to protect against negative energies and pollution and during astral travel. It is said that it changes color to warn of danger or illness. As well as helping us to feel grounded when undertaking spiritual work, turquoise is a powerful physical, emotional, mental, and spiritual healer that strengthens and regenerates the whole body.

Its many uses include providing pain relief and alleviating muscular and skeletal disorders, skin complaints, digestive problems, high blood pressure, asthma, fevers, and inflamed eyes.

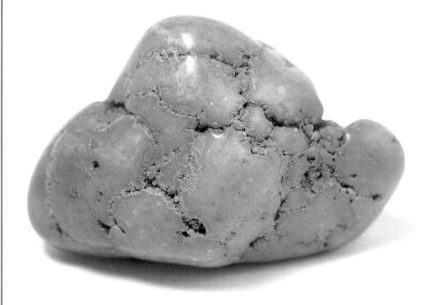

INDEX

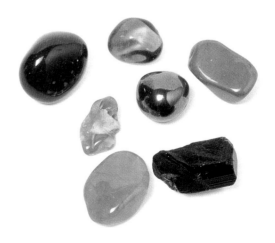

Useful Addresses

The address of the angel and crystal-healing website of Denise Whichello Brown, which gives details of workshops, crystals, and "aromacrystals," is www.angel-therapy.com

For information on workshops and training in complementary medicine under the personal supervision of Denise Whichello Brown, contact:

Beaumont College of Natural Medicine
M.W.B. Business Exchange
23 Hinton Road
Bournemouth
Dorset
BH1 2EF
United Kingdom
www.beaumontcollege.co.uk

Credits and Acknowledgements

My deepest love and gratitude to my dear husband, Garry, and children, Chloe and Thomas, for their patience and inspiration. Thanks also to Steve at Earthworks, who so patiently gave of his time.

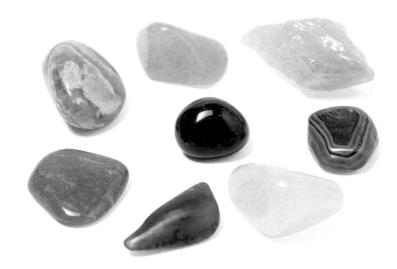